Managing heart f
in primary ca.

a practical guide

Managing heart failure in primary care
a practical guide

Martin R Cowie   Mike Kirby

BLADON
MEDICAL
PUBLISHING

© 2003 Bladon Medical Publishing
12 New Street, Chipping Norton, Oxfordshire
OX7 5LJ, UK

First published 2003

Always refer to the manufacturer's Prescribing Information
before prescribing drugs cited in this book.

British Library Cataloguing in Publication Data.
A catalogue record for this title is available from the British
Library

ISBN 1-904218-20-2

Martin R Cowie, Mike Kirby
Managing heart failure in primary care: a practical guide

Design and production:
Design Online Ltd, Oxford

Printed by
Talleres Gráficos Hostench s.a.
Venezuela, 87-93
Barcelona, Spain

Distributed by
Plymbridge Distributors Ltd,
Estover Road, Plymouth PL6 7PY, UK

Contents

Chapter 1

Heart failure: an overview

DEFINITION AND DIAGNOSIS

Heart failure is a clinical syndrome that results from any structural or functional cardiac disorder that impairs the ability of the heart to function as a pump. While the failing heart continues to function, it is unable to work as it should, particularly on exercise.

The syndrome is characterized by symptoms such as breathlessness and fatigue, both of which may limit exercise tolerance and signs such as fluid retention, which may lead to pulmonary congestion, raised jugular venous pressure and peripheral oedema. Patients do not usually exhibit all of the symptoms and signs at the same time. Both exercise intolerance and fluid retention may significantly reduce the patient's functional capacity and quality of life. Once patients have developed heart failure, they generally have a poor prognosis.

Heart failure may result from any disorder of the heart or major blood vessels, but the most common underlying problem is impairment of left ventricular function. This abnormality may be due to problems with contracting (systolic dysfunction) or relaxation and filling (diastolic dysfunction) of the ventricle or to both.

Despite being a result of cardiac dysfunction, heart failure is recognized and diagnosed principally on the basis of the symptoms and signs produced by the body's response to the cardiac abnormality. There is no single test that can be used for making the diagnosis. Heart failure is largely a clinical diagnosis that is based on a careful history and physical examination, with objective confirmation of the underlying cardiac abnormality securing the clinical diagnosis. A diagnosis of heart failure is not complete until its aetiology, severity and precipitating and exacerbating factors have been elucidated.[1,2]

EPIDEMIOLOGY

Epidemiological studies of heart failure have been complicated by differences in the diagnostic criteria and data collection, making national and international comparisons difficult. However, the available evidence suggests that the general population prevalence of heart failure is between three and 20 individuals per 1000, increasing to 30–130 per 1000 among those aged 75 years or older. The incidence of heart failure is generally in the range of one to five cases per 1000 population per year, rising steeply with age to more than 30 cases per 1000 population among those aged 75 years or older.[3,4]

Recent population-based studies conducted in the UK and elsewhere in Europe have shown that a general practitioner (GP) with a list of 2000 patients is likely to be caring for 20–30 patients with heart failure. Furthermore, there may be a similar number of patients with no

Figure 1.1   The incidence of heart failure in the Hillingdon Heart Study, London (1995–1996), by sex and age group.

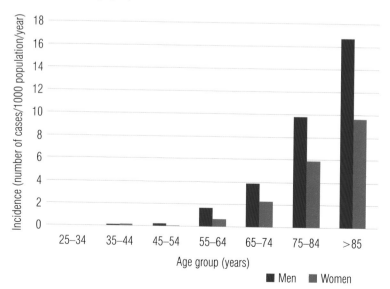

symptoms but significant cardiac disease (asymptomatic cardiac dysfunction). In addition, the average GP is likely to see approximately nine patients with suspected heart failure each year. Of these nine patients, three will have the diagnosis confirmed on further assessment.[5-9]

New cases of heart failure occur largely among the elderly. The median age at presentation in Northern Europe and the USA is approximately 75 years. The incidence rate is higher in men than in women (see Figure 1.1), chiefly as a result of coronary artery disease, which accounts for 60–70% of cases. However, as there are more elderly women than men in the population, the overall numbers are similar: there are approximately 475 000 men and 400 000 women aged 45 years and over living with confirmed or probable heart failure in the UK.[5-9]

THE HEALTH CARE BURDEN POSED BY HEART FAILURE

Heart failure is a multifactorial, multisystem disease that is complex to manage and, therefore, it poses a major burden to health services. The cost of illness studies from industrialized countries suggests that heart failure accounts for 1–2% of health care expenditure. In 1990/1991, the cost of chronic heart failure to the National Health Service (NHS) in the UK was estimated to be approximately £360 million. This rather conservative estimate represented 1% of the total NHS budget and 10% of the NHS expenditure on diseases of the circulatory system. Latest estimates have suggested that the cost of heart failure to the NHS had risen to £625 million by the year 2000.[9]

The burden posed by heart failure is likely to rise further and the prevalence of the syndrome is rising at an estimated 10% per annum. The reason for this rise is twofold.

1. The population is ageing. In the UK, people over 65 years currently number more than 9 million or 16% of the population, with over 1 million of those over the

age of 85 years. Figures from the Government Actuary's Department have suggested that the proportion of elderly people within the population will continue to grow at the expense of younger people within society. By the year 2051 there will be more than 15 million people aged over 65 years and as many as one in five of these will be over 85 years of age.[10]

2. Improved survival due to modern management of myocardial infarction is leaving more patients with a significantly damaged heart that is likely to fail at some point in the future.

As a result of the ageing of the population, the number of admissions for heart failure in the UK is projected to increase by more than 50% over the next 25 years, from 74 000 in 2000/2001 to 113 000 in 2026/2027.

A detailed breakdown shows that the cost of drugs and management in primary care accounts for a very small proportion of the overall total expenditure by the NHS on heart failure. The hospital costs of investigations and monitoring are considerably larger, but it is the cost associated with admission to hospital that drives the overall direct economic burden of heart failure to the NHS (see Figure 1.2).

Figure 1.2   Estimated direct economic cost of heart failure to the NHS in 2000 (McMurray *et al.*).

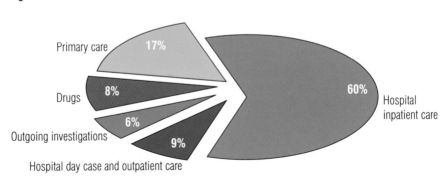

While the costs of illness studies are important to health service planners, they rarely give a true indication of the burden associated with any disease state either to society or to individual sufferers. Poorly controlled heart failure is disabling through its association with symptoms that impact directly on patients' ability to care for themselves, thus posing an additional burden on social services and family carers. The symptoms of heart failure also exert a major impact on all aspects of a patient's quality of life, probably more so than for any other chronic medical illness.[11] For example, depression is common among patients diagnosed with heart failure, but often goes unrecognized.

Hospitalization

Hospitalizations are common, frequent and often prolonged in patients with heart failure. The condition is known to account for approximately 5% of admissions to general medical and geriatric wards in UK hospitals. In 1990, the mean length of stay for an admission related to heart failure in an NHS hospital was 11.4 days on acute medical wards and 28.5 days on acute geriatric wards. Furthermore, once patients are discharged their readmission rates are as high as 33% within 12 months.[12–14]

Repeat hospitalization is particularly likely if deterioration of heart failure is not detected early enough. A prospective follow-up of incident cases of heart failure identified in a population-based survey in Bromley in south London showed that over half were subsequently hospitalized on one or more occasion over 19 months. Almost three-quarters of these hospitalizations were unplanned, with worsening heart failure accounting for approximately half.[15]

AETIOLOGY

Coronary artery disease is the most common cause of heart failure in Western societies, usually due to left ventricular systolic dysfunction. Other causes include high blood pressure, primary disease of the heart muscle (cardiomyopathy), valvular heart disease due to past rheumatic fever or other causes, congenital defects of the heart or great blood vessels, abnormal cardiac rhythms, alcoholic disease, pericardial disease and viral infection (see Table 1.1)

Full identification of the underlying cause is important to a diagnosis. In addition to having a direct impact upon the patient's treatment, in some cases heart failure can be reversed by treating the underlying causes. However, it is often difficult to ascertain the primary aetiology of heart failure in those patients with multiple potential causes.

Coronary artery disease, hypertension and other cardiovascular risk factors

Coronary artery disease is the principal cause of left ventricular systolic dysfunction in patients in developed societies. A history of hypertension is common in these

Table 1.1   Causes of heart failure

Causes	Characteristics
Coronary heart disease	Particularly myocardial infarction
Systemic or pulmonary hypertension	
Cardiomyopathies	Dilated, hypertrophic or restrictive/obliterative
Valvular disease	Usually mitral or aortic valve disease
Congenital heart disease	Particularly with chronic pressure or volume overload
Arrhythmias	Tachycardia (including atrial fibrillation) or bradycardia
Other causes	Pericardial disease (constrictive pericarditis and pericardial effusion), toxins (alcohol and anthracycline cytotoxics) and infections (HIV, coxsackie virus and Chagas' disease)

patients, but is rarely the sole cause of the patient's heart failure. In the Framingham Heart Study coronary artery disease or hypertension, either alone or in combination, was present in more than 90% of cases of heart failure.[16]

Population-based studies conducted in Europe have generally confirmed the Framingham Heart Study data. In the Hillingdon Heart Study coronary artery disease was the single most common aetiology (36%) identified in patients with a new diagnosis of heart failure. A history of hypertension was common (44%) among these patients.[5] In the Bromley Heart Study coronary artery disease was responsible for approximately half of all new cases of heart failure.[17]

The risk factors for coronary artery disease, such as smoking, hyperlipidaemia and diabetes, have also been found to be risk factors for the development of heart failure through their contributory effects to coronary artery disease. However, hypertension and diabetes are thought to contribute directly to the development of cardiac dysfunction.[18] Poorly controlled hypertension is known to cause left ventricular hypertrophy, while diabetes has also been shown to induce structural and functional changes in the myocardium.[19]

Hypertension may be a more important contributor to the development of heart failure among patients of African origin, while the increased prevalence of diabetes among south-eastern Asians is likely to make it a stronger contributor to the development of heart failure in this population.

Arrhythmias

Cardiac arrhythmias, particularly atrial fibrillation, frequently co-exist with heart failure and complicate its management. In the Hillingdon Heart Study 30% of patients presenting with new heart failure had atrial fibrillation. The presence of this arrhythmia is associated with a reduction in exercise capacity and a worse long-term prognosis.[20,21]

Ventricular arrhythmias are also more common in patients with heart failure and are a major cause of sudden death regardless of the cause of left ventricular systolic dysfunction.

Valvular disease

Valvular disease, particularly disease of the aortic and mitral valves, is an important cause of heart failure in developing nations. It is less important in the West. In the Framingham Heart Study 22% of men and 31% of women with heart failure of non-ischaemic aetiology had evidence of valvular disease. However, the contribution of valvular disease to the development of heart failure in the Framingham Heart Study cohort has declined dramatically.[16] Among the incident cases of heart failure reported in the Hillingdon Heart Study, valvular disease represented the primary aetiology in 11% of patients.[5]

CARDIOMYOPATHY

Primary diseases of heart muscle – those that are not secondary to coronary, hypertensive, valvular, congenital or pericardial abnormalities –are less common causes of heart failure. Nevertheless, these cardiomyopathies remain important for diagnostic purposes. The most important cardiomyopathies include the following.

- Dilated cardiomyopathy, where the predominant abnormality is dilatation of the left ventricle. It may be caused by a range of viral, bacterial or fungal infections, parasitic infections such as Chagas' disease and toxoplasmosis or connective tissue diseases such as systemic lupus erythematosus. In addition, chronic excessive alcohol consumption can exert a direct toxic effect upon the heart muscle (alcoholic cardiomyopathy), as can a number of prescribed drugs such as the anti-human immunodeficiency virus (HIV) agent zidovudine and anti-cancer drugs such as adriamycin, doxorubicin and trastuzumab. In some families an inherited gene defect may cause the development of dilated cardiomyopathy.

- Hypertrophic cardiomyopathy, which is a familial abnormality of the myocardial fibres that usually results in asymmetrical septal hypertrophy and which may be associated with aortic outflow obstruction

- Restrictive cardiomyopathy, where a stiff and poorly compliant ventricle results in diastolic dysfunction.

Strictly speaking, 'cardiomyopathy' was a term that was previously applied to cases where the cause of the myocardial dysfunction was unknown. With better understanding of the underlying genetic defects that can lead to some cases of cardiomyopathy, this term becomes less useful. Similarly, if the cause of the heart muscle damage is excessive alcohol consumption, then the label of cardiomyopathy may be less useful –some use the term 'alcoholic heart muscle disease' instead. Proper investigation of patients with heart failure should ensure that the aetiology of the condition is identified where possible. In a small minority of cases the aetiology cannot be established and the general term cardiomyopathy can be applied. It is bad practice to apply this label without investigating patients. This leaves the doctor open to the risk of missing a potentially reversible cause of cardiac damage.

Diastolic heart failure
When there is a strong clinical suspicion of heart failure due to the presence of appropriate signs and symptoms, but investigation reveals preserved left ventricular systolic function at rest and no valve or pericardial disease, diastolic heart failure is often presumed to be present. Diastolic dysfunction is most common in elderly patients, particularly in those with a history of systemic hypertension. In general, accurate diagnosis of the presence and aetiology of heart failure in elderly patients

may be more difficult due to the presence of other diseases and less enthusiasm for invasive investigation.

PATHOPHYSIOLOGY

Whatever the underlying cause of heart failure in any individual, the consequence is a decline in the pumping ability of the heart. This in turn initiates several compensatory mechanisms that affect the function of several different body systems. Therefore, chronic heart failure is ultimately a multisystem disorder.

Sympathetic nervous system activity is increased in a bid to maintain cardiac output and organ perfusion pressure by increasing the heart rate, myocardial contractility and peripheral vasoconstriction.[22] However, chronic sympathetic stimulation results in activation of a complex array of neurohormonal systems. The most fully understood system is probably the renin–angiotensin-aldosterone system: activation of this results in further vasoconstriction (through the action of angiotensin II), further elevation of plasma noradrenaline levels and salt and water retention and oedema. The effect is to increase the afterload on the heart, which leads to further deterioration in cardiac function.

In response to cardiac chamber stretch, the heart releases atrial natriuretic peptide and brain natriuretic peptide in an attempt to antagonize the effects of angiotensin II and lead to vasodilatation and increased urinary sodium excretion.

Other vasoactive peptides are also elevated in heart failure: endothelin is an extremely potent vasoconstrictor peptide secreted by vascular endothelial cells and produces further vasoconstriction and sodium retention.

In addition to effects on the heart, patients with chronic heart failure commonly show abnormalities in their skeletal muscle structure, metabolism and function, as well as a general reduction or wasting in muscle mass. These abnormalities contribute to the symptoms of tiredness and exercise intolerance generally reported by patients with chronic heart failure.

Recent research supports an inflammatory component to heart failure. The plasma levels of inflammatory cytokines such as tumour necrosis factor-α (TNFα) are elevated in patients with heart failure and correlate with disease severity, particularly in patients with cachexia.[23,24]

A better understanding of the pathophysiology of heart failure has opened up new therapeutic avenues, many of which are currently being explored. Some of these are outlined in Chapter 4.

PROGNOSIS

Once heart failure develops patients generally have a poor prognosis and mortality is high, particularly in the most severe forms of heart failure. In the Framingham Heart Study the survival rates were 57% at 1 year and 25% at 5 years in men and 64% at 1 year and 38% at 5 years in women.[25]

Figure 1.3 Cumulative survival of new (incident) cases of heart failure identified in the London Heart Failure Study, 1995–1998 (point estimates and 95% confidence intervals).

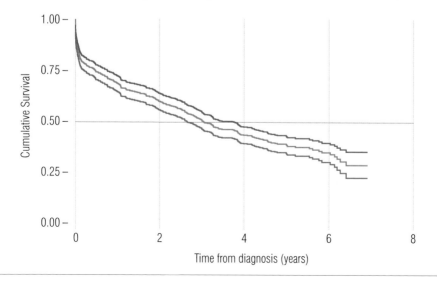

The population-based London Heart Failure Study confirmed this poor prognosis: in patients with new heart failure, mortality was high in the first few weeks after diagnosis (see Figure 1.3). Approximately 40% of patients had died within 12 months of diagnosis, while by 2 years 50% of patients had died.[5] As well as being elderly, most of these patients with newly diagnosed heart failure had considerable co-morbidity and a very high risk of subsequent hospitalization, particularly during the first months after diagnosis. This is considerably worse than reported from clinical trials, largely because of the highly selected nature of the patients entering such studies.

A diagnosis of heart failure appears to be more lethal than a diagnosis of cancer. Figures from the West Midlands Regional Cancer Registry (see Figure 1.4) have

Figure 1.4   Survival rates for heart failure and three common cancers (data from a joint report of the West Midlands Director of Public Health and West Midlands Regional Cancer Registry. Cancer and Health. Birmingham: West Midlands Regional Health Authority; 1995).

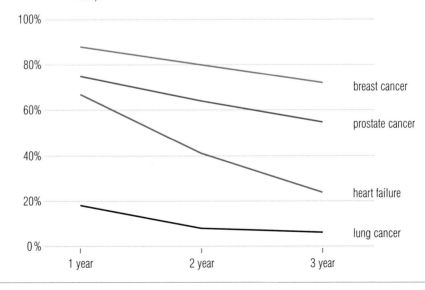

shown that the 1-year survival rates for patients diagnosed with heart failure are worse than for those diagnosed with breast, prostate and bladder cancer and similar to those diagnosed with cancer of the colon. Among common cancers only lung cancer has a poorer prognosis than heart failure.

Morbidity and quality of life
Heart failure is also associated with considerable morbidity. Compared to people without heart failure, those with heart failure are over three times as likely to have coronary heart disease and twice as likely to have diabetes. Symptoms of heart failure such as breathlessness can severely limit patients' physical activity and ability to perform everyday activities such as washing, dressing and walking between rooms. It is no surprise then that heart failure greatly impacts on patients' quality of life and that this impact becomes greater as the disease severity worsens.[26] One study suggested that heart failure causes more severe impairment of physical and social functioning and energy levels than chronic lung disease, arthritis or other cardiac conditions such as angina.[11]

ORGANIZATION OF CARE
Greater understanding of the pathophysiology of heart failure has led to advances in pharmacological management. Yet there appears to have been no substantial reduction in the morbidity and mortality associated with heart failure, suggesting that many patients are not managed optimally.[27,28]

Researchers have shown that those with special expertise often do not manage patients with heart failure, that effective therapies are often under-prescribed and that patients often have little understanding of their condition and its treatment. Therefore, the organization of heart failure care may be as important a contributor to the optimal care of patients with heart failure as purely medical interventions.

As experience of different disease management models

accumulates, it has become increasingly clear that the optimal management of heart failure requires an integrated multiprofessional approach. In particular, nurse-led care that includes a strong focus on patient education has been shown to reduce the rate of unplanned admissions and to increase the quality of life for patients with heart failure.[29–33]

Each patient with heart failure is unique in terms of the cause and course of their heart failure and in the way that they will approach their illness and its impact upon their lives. Nurse-led multidisciplinary care is more able to accept and respond to this than care based on the more traditional medical model.

AIMS OF MANAGEMENT

Over the last three decades treatment has moved away from a largely palliative approach to an approach that now focuses on (1) alleviating the symptoms, improving quality of life and prolonging survival and (2) preventing disease progression in patients with underlying structural cardiac abnormalities.

In patients with previous myocardial infarction or hypertension prevention of disease progression is achieved by slowing or reversing left ventricular remodelling and thereby slowing, halting or even reversing the deterioration in left ventricular systolic dysfunction. This approach also holds out the hope of stemming the tide of incident heart failure through appropriate preventive approaches among those groups within the population most at risk of developing left ventricular dysfunction. Preventive efforts should be aimed at the treatment of hypertension and diabetes and management of athero-sclerotic disease and also at the control of conditions that may cause cardiac injury, such as smoking and alcohol abuse. In addition, cardioprotective therapy (such as angiotensin-converting enzyme (ACE) inhibitors and beta blockers) should be considered for all patients who have suffered a myocardial infarction, irrespective of whether they have symptoms of heart failure. Echocardiography is likely to reveal that many such patients will already have suffered damage to their left ventricle.

This book provides a summary of best practice in the diagnosis and management of heart failure, including the various therapeutic strategies currently available. Key points are illustrated by case studies. Further sources of information and guidance are referenced throughout the text and at the end of the book.

Case Study

A typical heart failure patient

Harold Brown, who retired 3 years ago, is an active 68-year-old man who suffered an anterior myocardial infarction 10 years ago. Although he recovered well he has since suffered from mild hypertension, which his GP has controlled with bendrofluazide. Following the advice of his GP, Harold gave up smoking after his infarct and now watches his diet quite closely as a means of managing his blood cholesterol. Although he is not obese, he is somewhat overweight.

He recently presented to his GP, who had not seen him for several years, complaining that he gets breathless when playing golf and also gets puffed by the time he reaches the top of the stairs at home. His ankles are slightly swollen by the end of the day, but they seem to go down again by the morning.

The GP examined Harold and confirmed the presence of dependent oedema. His blood pressure (on treatment) was 150/86 mmHg. An electrocardiogram showed sinus rhythm, but with deep Q waves in V1–V3, in keeping with his previous anterior myocardial infarction. The chest X-ray showed mild cardiomegaly and upper lobe venous blood diversion. Suspecting heart failure, the GP organized an open-access echocardiogram. This confirmed a slightly dilated left ventricle, the anterior wall of which did not move, suggesting dead tissue. It also showed

moderately impaired systolic function of the left ventricle (ejection fraction 28%).

The most likely cause of Harold's symptoms was heart failure due to coronary heart disease with a possible contribution from his hypertension and his weight problem. Therefore, the GP changed his bendrofluazide to a low dose of frusemide (20 mg once daily) and started him on an ACE inhibitor (lisinopril). Harold noticed a marked improvement in his breathlessness within 1 week, but the GP was insistent on increasing the dose of lisinopril gradually. He also wanted to introduce a beta blocker within 2 months, once the right dose of lisinopril had been reached. The GP checked Harold's urea and electrolytes when he started the lisinopril; these were normal and remained so each time he increased the dose.

The GP explained to Harold and his wife, who was also present at the consultation, that Harold had heart failure, which was probably due to his coronary heart disease, which had also caused his earlier heart attack. He explained that, although the drugs he was prescribing would help, Harold also had to help himself by getting his weight down towards the normal weight for his height and by continuing to take physical activity.

He also mentioned that subsequently he might need to alter his diuretic dosages if the fluid retention became a problem again.

REFERENCES

1. Hunt SA, Baker DW, Chin MH. *ACC/AHA Guidelines for the Evaluation and Management of Chronic Heart Failure in the Adult. A Report of the American College of Cardiology/American Heart Association Task Force on Practice Guidelines (Committee to Revise the 1995 Guidelines for the Evaluation and Management of Heart Failure)*.

2. The Task Force for the Diagnosis and Treatment of Chronic Heart Failure, European Society of Cardiology. Guidelines for the diagnosis and treatment of chronic heart failure. *Eur Heart J* 2001; **22**: 1527–60.

3. Cowie MR, Mosterd A, Wood DA *et al*. The epidemiology of heart failure. *Eur Heart J* 1997; **18**: 208–15.

4. Ho KK, Pinsky JL, Kannel WB, Levy D. The epidemiology of heart failure: the Framingham Study. *J Am Coll Cardiol* 1993; **22**: 6–13A.

5. Cowie MR, Wood DA, Coats AJS *et al*. Incidence and aetiology of heart failure: a population-based study. *Eur Heart J* 1999; **20**: 421–8.

6. Mosterd A, Hoes AW, De Bruyne MC *et al*. Prevalence of heart failure and left ventricular dysfunction in the general population; The Rotterdam Study. *Eur Heart J* 1999; **20**: 447–55.

7. Davies M, Hobbs F, Davis R *et al*. Prevalence of left-ventricular systolic dysfunction and heart failure in the Echocardiographic Heart of England Screening Study: a population based study. *Lancet* 2001; **358**: 439–44.

8. McDonagh TA, Morrison CE, Lawrence A *et al*. Symptomatic and asymptomatic left-ventricular systolic dysfunction in an urban population. *Lancet* 1997; **350**: 829–33.

9. Petersen S, Rayner M. *British Heart Foundation Statistics Database 2002. Coronary Morbidity Supplement – Heart Failure*. London: British Heart Foundation; 2002.

10. Emmerson C, Frayne C, Goodman A. *Pressures in UK Healthcare: Challenges for the NHS*. Institute for Fiscal Studies; 2000.

11. Stewart AL, Greenfield S, Hays RD *et al*. Functional status and well-being of patients with chronic conditions. Results from the Medical Outcomes Study. *JAMA* 1989; **262**: 907–13.

12. Parameshwar J, Poole-Wilson PA, Sutton GC. Heart failure in a district general hospital. *J R Coll Phys Lond* 1992; **26**: 139–42.

13. McMurray J, Hart W, Rhodes G. An evaluation of the cost of heart failure to the National Health Service in the UK. *Br J Med Econ* 1993; **6**: 99–110.

14. McMurray J, McDonagh T, Morrison CE *et al*. Trends in hospitalization for heart failure in Scotland 1980–1990. *Eur Heart J* 1993; **14**: 1158–62.

15. Cowie MR, Fox KF, Wood DA *et al*. Hospitalization of patients with heart failure: a population-based study. *Eur Heart J* 2002; **23**: 877–85.

16. Kannel WB, Ho K, Thomas T. Changing epidemiological features of cardiac failure. *Br Heart J* 1994; **72**(Suppl): S3–9.

17. Fox KF, Cowie MR, Wood DA *et al*. Coronary artery disease as the cause of incident heart failure in the population. *Eur Heart J* 2001; **22**: 228–36.

18. Solang L, Malmberg K, Ryden L. Diabetes mellitus and congestive heart failure. Further knowledge needed. *Eur Heart J* 1999; **20**: 789–95.

19. Vasan RS, Larson MG, Benjamin EJ, Evans JC, Reiss CK, Levy D. Congestive heart failure in subjects with normal versus reduced left ventricular ejection fraction: prevalence and mortality in a population-based cohort. *J Am Coll Cardiol* 1999; **33**: 1948–55.

20. Stevenson WG, Stevenson LW. Atrial fibrillation in heart failure (editorial). *N Engl J Med* 1999; **341**: 910–11.

21. Dries DL, Exner DV, Gersh BJ *et al.* Atrial fibrillation is associated with an increased risk for mortality and heart failure progression in patients with asymptomatic and symptomatic left ventricular systolic dysfunction: a retrospective analysis of the SOLVD trials. Studies of Left Ventricular Dysfunction. *J Am Coll Cardiol* 1998; **32**: 695–703.
22. Katz AM. Heart failure in 2001: a prophecy revisited. *Am J Cardiol* 2001; **87**: 1383–6.
23. McMurray J, Abdullah I, Dargie HJ, Shapiro D. Increased concentrations of tumour necrosis factor in 'cachectic' patients with severe chronic heart failure. *Br Heart J* 1991; **66**: 356–8.
24. Mann DL, Young JB. Basic mechanisms in congestive heart failure. Recognizing the role of proinflammatory cytokines. *Chest* 1994; **105**(3): 897–904.
25. Ho KK, Anderson KM, Kannel WB *et al.* Survival after the onset of congestive heart failure in Framingham Heart Study subjects. *Circulation* 1993; **88**: 107–15.
26. Hobbs FDR, Kenkre JE, Roalfe AK *et al.* Impact of heart failure and left ventricular systolic dysfunction on quality of life: a cross-sectional study comparing chronic cardiac and medical disorders and a representative adult population. *Eur J Heart Failure* (in press).
27. Ashton CM. Care of patients with failing hearts: evidence for failures in clinical practice and health services research. *J Gen Intern Med* 1999; **14**: 138–40.
28. Chin MH, Goldman L. Factors contributing to the hospitalization of patients with congestive heart failure. *Am J Public Hlth* 1997; **87**: 643–8.
29. Rich MW, Beckham V, Wittenberg C *et al.* A multidisciplinary intervention to prevent the readmission of elderly patients with congestive heart failure. *N Engl J Med* 1995; **333**: 1190–5.
30. Stewart S, Marley JE, Horowitz JD. Effects of a multidisciplinary, home-based intervention on unplanned readmissions and survival among patients with chronic congestive heart failure: a randomised controlled study. *Lancet* 1999; **354**: 1077–83.
31. Stewart S, Vandenbroek AJ, Pearson S, Horowitz JD. Prolonged beneficial effects of a home-based intervention on unplanned readmissions and mortality among patients with congestive heart failure. *Arch Intern Med* 1999; **159**: 257–61.
32. Cline CMJ, Israelsson BYA, Willenheimer RB *et al.* Cost effective management programme for heart failure reduces hospitalisation. *Heart* 1998; **80**: 442–6.
33. Blue L, Lang E, McMurray JJV *et al.* Randomised controlled trial of specialist nurse intervention in heart failure. *BMJ* 2001; **323**: 715–18.

Chapter 2

Diagnosing and investigating heart failure

Patients with heart failure usually present with symptoms such as breathlessness, fatigue and fluid retention. Because these symptoms are relatively non-specific, they alone cannot be relied upon for making a diagnosis: good clinical skills with history taking and a careful physical examination need to be supplemented by further investigative tests. Diagnosis requires consideration of:

- the underlying abnormality of the heart
- the severity of the syndrome
- the aetiology
- the precipitating and exacerbating factors
- concomitant disease relevant to management
- the likely prognosis.

Identification of any reversible cause of heart damage is particularly important. Cardiac function can be severely impaired by arrhythmias or myocardial ischaemia, even in patients without major permanent cardiac dysfunction. Treatment of these problems may have a dramatic impact on the patient. Myocardial ischaemia, changes in valvular regurgitation, pulmonary embolism, infection, arrhythmia (most notably atrial fibrillation), renal dysfunction, anaemia, thyroid disease, the side-effects of drug therapy (particularly non-steroidal anti-inflammatory drugs (NSAIDs)) and excessive fluid, sodium or alcohol intake may cause or exacerbate the heart failure syndrome in patients with cardiac damage and chronic heart failure. If the primary disorder is valvular then in some cases the heart failure can be cured by valve repair or replacement (see Chapter 5).

SIGNS AND SYMPTOMS OF HEART FAILURE

Patients with heart failure may present with a number of symptoms. The most common of these are breathlessness, fatigue, exercise intolerance and fluid retention, particularly ankle swelling. However, patients may also present with other symptoms that may include nocturia, anorexia, abdominal bloating and discomfort, constipation and cerebral symptoms such as confusion, dizziness and memory impairment.

The degree of exertion required to elicit breathlessness or other limiting symptoms may be used for grading the severity of heart failure into one of four functional classes using the New York Heart Association (NYHA) classification for heart failure (see Table 2.1).

It is important for clinicians to remember that the severity of the symptoms does not necessarily indicate the severity of the underlying heart problem: some patients with severe damage to the heart will have only mild symptoms, while those with minor damage to the heart may suffer severe symptoms. In addition, the severity of the symptoms tends to fluctuate, irrespective of treatment. However, in general, patients' functional class does tend to deteriorate over time. The NYHA classification may be used for monitoring the effects of treatment. Changes in medication and diet can affect patients' functional capacity in the absence of any measurable change in heart function.

Table 2.1   The NYHA classification of heart failure

Class	Definition
Class I	Ordinary physical exercise does not cause undue fatigue or breathlessness
Class II	Slight limitation of physical activity: comfortable at rest, but ordinary physical activity, for example minor activities such as climbing a flight of stairs, getting dressed or doing housework, results in fatigue, palpitations or breathlessness
Class III	Marked limitation of physical activity: comfortable at rest, but symptoms such as breathlessness occur when walking on a flat surface
Class IV	Unable to carry out any physical activity without discomfort: symptoms occur even at rest with increased discomfort with any physical activity

BEWARE OF ALTERNATIVE DIAGNOSES

Many other conditions may present with symptoms similar to those of heart failure and this at least partially explains why surveys have shown that less than one-half of patients in whom a general practitioner (GP) suspects heart failure have this diagnosis confirmed on further investigation.[1-3]

Obesity is commonly misdiagnosed as heart failure, particularly in women, because it may cause breathlessness, fatigue and ankle swelling.

Pulmonary embolic disease, pulmonary disease such as fibrosing alveolitis, bilateral renal artery stenosis, intrinsic renal or hepatic disease, anaemia and thyroid disease may all mimic heart failure or, in the case of anaemia and thyroid disease, can aggravate symptoms in a patient with heart failure.

Elderly patients in particular are likely to have a number of concomitant medical problems or to be taking drugs that can cause diagnostic confusion. Ankle swelling may for instance be caused by treatment with a dihydropyridine calcium channel blocker. Similarly, NSAIDs may result in sodium and water retention.

ALWAYS START WITH THE HISTORY

The symptoms of heart failure – breathlessness, ankle swelling and fatigue – may be difficult to interpret, particularly in elderly or obese patients. Therefore, before a diagnosis of heart failure can be considered in any patient who presents with these symptoms, the GP should first take a careful and detailed history and undertake a full clinical examination.

The history should extend beyond the immediate cardiac problem, particularly in elderly patients in whom co-morbidities will be common. Diseases of the peripheral vasculature and organs such as the kidney and lungs may affect both the diagnosis and choice of treatment. For instance, in patients with benign prostatic hypertrophy a vigorous diuresis may precipitate acute urinary retention and in those with reversible airways obstruction a beta blocker will be contraindicated.

The clinical signs of heart failure should be assessed carefully by examining the cardiovascular system and lung fields carefully. It is important to look for:

- murmurs and thrills as a sign of valve disease
- a displaced apex beat, which may be a sign of left ventricular enlargement
- a bounding apex beat, which is a sign of left ventricular hypertrophy.

Lung crackles are common in the elderly, but may point towards heart failure if they are fine in nature, extend beyond the bases and do not clear on coughing. A raised jugular venous pressure is of most predictive value: this indicates raised right atrial pressure and a high likelihood of heart failure in a patient with breathlessness. Dependent oedema is also a useful clinical sign, although it does not have as high a predictive value as a raised jugular venous pressure. Tachycardia, a third heart sound and a displaced apex beat are also suggestive of underlying cardiac abnormality.

The more clinical signs present, the greater the likelihood of heart failure. While a diagnosis can be made with greater confidence in the presence of multiple signs and symptoms, further assessment and investigative tests are always required in order to identify the underlying functional abnormalities before a full diagnosis can be made with confidence.

Treatment with a diuretic may dramatically reduce both the symptoms and clinical signs of fluid retention and may make a diagnosis more difficult. In some circumstances such therapy is required because of the severity of the symptoms and it should not be withheld just because of a desire to make a 'full-house' textbook diagnosis.

USEFUL DIAGNOSTIC INVESTIGATIONS

Symptoms and signs are important in alerting the GP to the possibility that a patient may have heart failure.

However, this clinical suspicion of heart failure must be confirmed by more objective tests, particularly those aimed at assessing cardiac function.

A patient with suspected heart failure should have the following investigations:

- a 12-lead electrocardiogram (ECG)

- a chest radiograph,

- blood biochemistry

- cardiac imaging, usually by transthoracic echo-cardiography

- plasma B-type natriuretic peptide (BNP) or N-terminal pro-BNP (NTproBNP).

These tests will not only help confirm the clinical diagnosis but will also help exclude other pathologies that may masquerade as heart failure, such as renal failure or severe anaemia. They may also identify co-morbidities that can influence management.

The measurement of plasma natriuretic peptides may be very useful in excluding heart failure; patients with a normal blood concentration of BNP or NTproBNP are unlikely to have heart failure and it would be sensible to explore other diagnoses (see below).

Local protocols and service availability will determine the order in which tests are carried out. Figure 2.1 illustrates a proposed algorithm for the diagnosis of a patient with suspected heart failure.

Twelve-lead ECG

Patients with heart failure frequently show electrocardiographic changes; a completely normal ECG is unlikely in a patient with chronic heart failure due to left ventricular systolic dysfunction. However, the presence of an abnormality in an ECG does not necessarily confirm a diagnosis of heart failure and further investigation is required: minor changes in ECGs are almost universal in the very elderly.

The presence of anterior Q waves and a left bundle branch block in patients with ischaemic heart disease are good predictors of systolic dysfunction. ECG signs of left atrial overload ('P mitrale') or left ventricular hypertrophy may also be associated with left ventricular dysfunction.

An ECG is particularly important for detecting atrial fibrillation or flutter and, sometimes, ventricular arrhythmia as a causal or contributory factor to a patient's heart failure. If the history suggests paroxysmal arrhythmia a 24-hour ECG recording may be valuable.

Figure 2.1   Algorithm for the diagnosis of a patient with suspected heart failure. With regard to imaging by echocardiography, alternative methods of imaging the heart should be considered when transthoracic Doppler and two-dimensional-echocardiography produce a poor image: the alternative method may be transoesophageal echocardiography, radionuclide imaging or cardiac magnetic resonance imaging (MRI).

Suspected heart failure
because of history, symptoms and signs

▼

Blood tests: full blood count, urea and electrolytes, creatinine, thyroid function tests, liver function tests, glucose & lipids
Urinalysis: sugar, blood & protein

▼

Assess presence of cardiac disease by **ECG, chest X-ray and natriuretic peptides** (BNP or NTproBNP)

▼ **All normal**
Heart Failure very unlikely

▼ **Abnormal**

▼

Imaging by echocardiography

▼ **Normal**
Heart Failure unlikely, but if diagnostic doubt persists consider 'diastolic heart failure' and referral for specialist assessment

▼ **Abnormal**
Assess Heart Failure severity, aetiology, precipitating and exacerbating factors and type of cardiac dysfunction

Chest radiograph

Although a chest radiograph should be part of the initial diagnostic work-up in suspected heart failure it rarely provides conclusive evidence for the presence of heart failure. However, it may be useful in detecting raised left atrial pressure with upper lobe venous blood diversion and interstitial or alveolar pulmonary oedema. Cardiac enlargement may also be suspected (by, for example, a cardiothoracic ratio of >0.50) although this may be misleading, particularly in the elderly and an echocardiogram is much better at assessing cardiac chamber dimensions (and function). Importantly, acute heart failure and diastolic heart failure may occur even with a completely normal-sized heart. A chest radiograph may uncover other diagnoses, for example a lung tumour, pneumothorax or pneumonia and this alone makes the chest radiograph useful in the investigation of patients with breathlessness.

Cardiac imaging: echocardiography

Cardiac imaging, usually by transthoracic Doppler and echocardiography, should be performed wherever possible when a diagnosis of heart failure is being considered.

Echocardiography is rapid, safe and can provide detailed information about the structure and function of the cardiac chambers, valves and pericardium. It is important that someone skilled in this investigation uses a high-resolution machine for performing the scan. The clinical value of this test is maximized when the clinical history and the reason for the request is clear to the echocardiographer.

One frequently quoted measure of left ventricular systolic function is the ejection fraction. This gives some indication of how well the ventricle contracts, although the variation in results from one echocardiographer to another and from one scan to another is not insignificant. The most useful echocardiography reports will not only provide technical information on the structure and function of the cardiac chambers, valves and pericardium but will also set this in a clinical context and help the GP to make informed decisions about therapy.

Diastolic function is difficult to assess without resorting to haemodynamic measurements at cardiac catheterization. Various measurements can be made on a Doppler echocardiography, but their interpretation can be difficult, particularly in the very elderly or in those in atrial fibrillation. If diastolic heart failure is suspected then a specialist assessment of the scan and the patient should be considered.

Alternative methods of imaging the heart may need to be considered when echocardiography produces a poor image. This is more likely if a patient has chronic obstructive lung disease or is obese. Alternative imaging methods may include radionuclide angiography or cardiac MRI. Specialist referral will almost certainly be required in these instances.

OPEN ACCESS TO ECHOCARDIOGRAPHY

The key issue regarding echocardiography in the UK is access. Many patients with heart failure present initially to their GP, yet echocardiography has until recently only been available through specialist referral to hospital-based specialists.

Open access echocardiography services have helped to speed up the objective confirmation of underlying cardiac dysfunction in patients with suspected heart failure. These services work best where there are clear guidelines for requesting studies, which should only be performed on high-resolution equipment by experienced operators. A cardiologist's interpretation of the scan maximizes the value of the test, but in the future GPs with a special interest and training in cardiac imaging may well provide this interpretation with recourse to a specialist only for complex cases. Accreditation may be necessary and may present something of a stumbling block to the wider use of echocardiography in primary care.

Plasma natriuretic peptides (BNP and NTproBNP)

Plasma concentrations of certain natriuretic peptides, which are produced by myocardial tissue in response to cardiac stretch or 'strain', can be helpful in ruling out a diagnosis of heart failure.

A number of clinical and epidemiological studies have shown that decreasing left ventricular function leads to an increasing plasma concentration of atrial natriuretic peptide, BNP and its co-secreted but inactive partner NTproBNP. Patients with heart failure have grossly elevated circulating levels of BNP (and NTproBNP). Studies in both primary and secondary care suggest that, in those patients in whom the plasma concentrations of BNP or NTproBNP are normal, other causes of dyspnoea and associated symptoms should be considered, as heart failure is unlikely. In those patients in whom the plasma concentrations of BNP or NTproBNP are elevated, further investigations, such as echocardiography or other tests of cardiac function, should be considered.[3]

The role of natriuretic peptides will expand in the future. They may have a role in screening strategies for individuals at high risk of heart failure (such as those with coronary artery disease, hypertension or diabetes) and using serial outpatient measurement for adjusting heart failure therapy may improve the clinical outcome over that found when conventional clinical assessment alone is used.[4]

Blood biochemistry and urinalysis

A number of laboratory haematological and biochemical investigations are recommended in the routine diagnostic evaluation of patients with symptoms that may be due to heart failure. These should include a complete blood count (haemoglobin, leukocytes and platelets), serum electrolytes, creatinine, glucose and hepatic enzymes, thyroid and liver function tests and possibly also blood lipids. Urinalysis will also help assist in the detection of renal dysfunction and diabetes mellitus.

These investigations should contribute to the building up of a more complete picture of the individual patient's disease. The following should be taken into account.

1. Anaemia may exacerbate pre-existing heart failure or lead to a syndrome resembling heart failure (symptoms of breathlessness and fatigue with fluid retention).

2. A raised haematocrit suggests that breathlessness may be due to pulmonary disease, cyanotic congenital heart disease or a pulmonary arteriovenous malformation.

3. Heart failure and renal dysfunction often coincide because of the underlying disease, such as diabetes and hypertension or as a consequence of impaired kidney perfusion. It is important to remember that elevated serum creatinine may be caused by primary renal disease, which may induce all the features of 'heart failure' by volume overload. Where there is diagnostic doubt, specialist referral is advisable. Hyponatraemia and renal dysfunction in the setting of heart failure indicate a bad prognosis.

4. Urinalysis is useful in detecting proteinuria and glycosuria, indicating the possibility of underlying renal problems or diabetes mellitus, which may contribute to or complicate heart failure.

5. Heart failure with rapid atrial fibrillation may be due to thyrotoxicosis and these may be the presenting features of thyrotoxicosis in the elderly. Hypothyroidism may also present as heart failure.

6. Liver function tests. These may be abnormal due to hepatic congestion secondary to heart failure. Alternatively, derangement may indicate primary liver disease, which can cause fluid retention and lead to diagnostic confusion. Excessive alcohol consumption may also be suggested by raised blood g-GT concentrations.

Pulmonary function testing
Pulmonary function tests provide little additional diagnostic information to that provided by symptoms,

signs and other non-invasive tests, but they can be useful in excluding respiratory causes of breathlessness.

Cardiopulmonary exercise testing

Cardiopulmonary exercise testing (with analysis of carbon dioxide production and oxygen consumption) has only a limited value in the diagnosis of heart failure and is not usually performed. A normal maximal exercise test in a patient not receiving treatment for heart failure may be useful for excluding heart failure as a diagnosis. However, cardiopulmonary exercise testing can provide objective information on the patient's functional ability and may be useful in estimating the patient's prognosis.

WHEN TO REFER FOR A SPECIALIST OPINION

In most cases the investigations outlined above will rapidly confirm a clinical diagnosis of heart failure. However, where the diagnosis is uncertain the patient should be referred for more specialist assessment. If the symptoms are very severe or if the patient is very unwell, then urgent admission for assessment and treatment may be essential.

Specialist input is most likely to be worthwhile in patients with angina, atrial fibrillation, valve disease, cardiomyopathy, congenital heart disease and in pregnancy. It is also essential in circumstances where specialist interventions such as revascularization, valve replacement, heart transplantation or cardiac assist devices might be considered.

Some patients with heart failure, particularly among the elderly, have no obvious valvular or systolic impairment of the heart and are assumed to have 'diastolic' abnormalities accounting for the syndrome. This is more likely if there is a history of hypertension. A definitive diagnosis can only be made at cardiac catheterization, but the echocardiogram may give some pointers towards this diagnosis. A specialist opinion may assist in firming up the diagnosis. The appropriate treatment for these patients is not known, but several clinical trials are ongoing. In the meantime such patients are usually treated with angiotensin-converting enzyme (ACE) inhibitors and diuretics.

LINKING DIAGNOSIS TO TREATMENT

Once the patient has been fully evaluated and a diagnosis of heart failure has been confirmed, the focus of clinical attention must switch to management with the aim of providing symptomatic relief for the patient while also preventing further deterioration in cardiac function.

Table 2.2 shows the management outline recommended by the European Society of Cardiology.[5]

Table 2.2 The European Society of Cardiology's recommended management process

Management outline

1.	Establish that the patient has heart failure
2.	Ascertain presenting features: pulmonary oedema, breathlessness on exertion, fatigue and peripheral oedema
3.	Assess the severity of symptoms
4.	Determine the aetiology of heart failure
5.	Identify precipitating and exacerbating factors
6.	Identify concomitant diseases relevant to heart failure and its management
7.	Estimate the prognosis
8.	Anticipate complications
9.	Counsel patient and relatives
10.	Choose appropriate management
11.	Monitor progress and manage accordingly

The management of patients with heart failure includes lifestyle changes and pharmacological therapy. Surgery or other invasive procedures will be required in some patients. The currently available types of management within each category are outlined in Table 2.3 and explained more fully in the following chapters.

Table 2.3   Treatment options open to patients with heart failure

Non-pharmacological management

General advice and measures

Exercise and exercise training

Pharmacological therapy

Diuretics

ACE inhibitors

Angiotensin II receptor blockers

Beta blockers

Aldosterone receptor antagonists

Cardiac glycosides

Anti-arrhythmic agents

Other vasodilator agents (nitrates/hydralazine)

Anticoagulation

Other intravenous/oral inotropic agents

Investigational therapies

Devices and surgery

Revascularization (catheter interventions and surgery) and other forms of surgery

Pacemakers

Implantable cardioverter defibrillators

Heart transplantation, ventricular assist devices and artificial hearts

Ultrafiltration and haemodialysis

Case Studies

Heart failure complicated by ischaemia and hibernation

Mavis West, a 67-year-old woman, presented to her GP complaining of breathlessness when she climbed the stairs or carried heavy shopping and also of occasional discomfort across the chest usually related to exertion. She had always had puffy ankles, but thought they were now slightly worse.

Mavis was a diet-controlled diabetic who was slightly overweight, but not on any kind of treatment from her GP. She was a smoker, but stopped 10 years ago. However, she did have a family history of coronary artery disease in her male relatives.

The GP performed an ECG, which showed ST depression in leads V4–V6 and referred her for a chest X-ray and echocardiogram. The chest X-ray showed a normal-sized heart but some interstitial shadowing, while the echocardiogram revealed a mildly dilated left ventricle with overall mildly reduced systolic function (ejection fraction 35%) and the lateral wall less active than the remainder of the left ventricle (lateral hypokinesia).

The GP suspected that Mavis had both heart failure and angina and started her on a low-dose diuretic, aspirin and oral isosorbide mononitrate and gave her a GTN spray. He also referred her for an urgent cardiology assessment.

In response to therapy and before she saw the consultant, her breathlessness was somewhat better although her ankle swelling was little changed and the GTN spray had relieved her chest discomfort. The consultant organized an exercise test, which she stopped at 6 min due to breathlessness and chest tightness, with marked ST depression in V4–V6. The cardiologist then organized a coronary angiogram, which revealed three-vessel coronary artery disease. He confirmed impaired left ventricular function and referred her for coronary artery bypass surgery.

In the meantime she was started on low-dose carvedilol under hospital supervision, which was increased at 2-weekly intervals until her bypass, which occurred 2 months after her first presentation to the GP.

After recovering from the bypass surgery, she no longer experienced breathlessness or chest pain. Follow-up echocardiograms revealed improvement in her left ventricular function with a marked reduction in her heart size, due to 'hibernating' muscle regaining the ability to contract.

Heart failure complicated by atrial fibrillation

Albert Shufflethwaite, a 78-year-old man with a history of well-controlled hypertension on bendrofluazide, presented to his GP with palpitation and breathlessness. His palpitation was most noticeable when he tried to sleep on his left-hand side and when he tried to push a trolley around the supermarket. His ankles were also prone to becoming increasingly swollen, particularly by the end of the day. On examination the GP noticed his swollen ankles and his irregular pulse, at approximately 100–110 beats/min, with an obviously raised jugular venous pressure at 6 cm. She suspected atrial fibrillation and heart failure and changed Albert's

Case Studies

Heart failure complicated by atrial fibrillation continued

diuretic to a loop diuretic. She also started therapy with an ACE inhibitor.

An ECG confirmed atrial fibrillation, so the GP arranged for an urgent echocardiogram and urea and electrolytes and was concerned regarding the need for initiating anticoagulation because of the risk of thromboembolism.

After telephone consultation with the cardiac unit, it was agreed that, provided the blood tests (including INR and liver function tests) were normal, the patient should be started on warfarin with an early review in the cardiac clinic for consideration of cardioversion. In the meantime the GP was advised to start Albert on digoxin.

The patient was seen in the cardiac clinic the following week, at which point he was much less breathless, though still in atrial fibrillation, but

now on anticoagulation. The echocardiogram showed mildly dilated left and right atria and mildly impaired left ventricular systolic function, although the irregularity of the heartbeat made assessment slightly difficult.

The consultant saw Albert and his wife and advised that he undergo DC cardioversion under a general anaesthetic, which was performed the following week, returning him to sinus rhythm.

Albert's symptoms have now completely resolved. The decision was made to maintain him on warfarin for 3 months in case of relapse to atrial fibrillation and to continue therapy with an ACE inhibitor. Repeat echocardiography in sinus rhythm revealed only mildly impaired left ventricular systolic dysfunction and slightly enlarged atria.

Heart failure due to diastolic dysfunction

Hyacinth Adams, a 56-year-old, non-smoking Afro-Caribbean woman with a long history of difficult to control hypertension, presented to her GP with cough and breathlessness, which kept her awake at night. The GP elicited a history of orthopnoea and paroxysmal nocturnal dyspnoea and undertook a series of investigations. The ECG showed sinus rhythm with voltage criteria for left ventricular hypertrophy, while the chest X-ray showed a heart at the upper limit of normal size, but with interstitial lung shadowing. Renal function revealed a urea of 10.1 mmol/l and a creatinine of 180 μmol/l. The GP diagnosed heart failure and initiated treatment with a diuretic pending the results of an echocardiogram and blood tests.

When the echocardiogram results came through they showed marked left ventricular hypertrophy with good systolic function, but an enlarged left atrium and Doppler indices reported as being in keeping with diastolic dysfunction. Hyacinth's blood pressure at this point was 180/90 mmHg, for which she was on amlodipine and low-dose enalapril. The GP added in bendrofluazide and increased the dose of the ACE inhibitor while checking her urea and electrolytes carefully. He also referred her to the hospital hypertension clinic for fine-tuning of her hypertension and diastolic heart failure.

REFERENCES

1. Wheeldon NM, MacDonald TM, Flucker CJ *et al.* Echocardiography in chronic heart failure in the community. *Q J Med* 1993; **86**: 17–23.
2. Remes J, Miettinen H, Reunanen A, Pyorala K. Validity of clinical diagnosis of heart failure in primary health care. *Eur Heart J* 1991; **12**: 315–21.
3. Cowie MR, Struthers AD, Wood DA *et al.* Value of natriuretic peptides in assessment of patients with possible new heart failure in primary care. *Lancet* 1997; **350**: 1349–53.
4. Cowie MR, Mendez GF. BNP and congestive heart failure. *Prog Cardiovasc Disease* 2002; **44**: 293–321.
5. The Task Force for the Diagnosis and Treatment of Chronic Heart Failure, European Society of Cardiology. Guidelines for the diagnosis and treatment of chronic heart failure. *Eur Heart J* 2001; **22**: 1527–60.

Chapter 3

General management

After a proper diagnosis of heart failure is made and explained to the patient management should begin with the provision of general advice and a full discussion of the role that the patient and carer can play in managing the condition.

Many patients assume that 'heart failure' means 'cardiac arrest'. It is important to explain to the patient and to their close relatives that heart failure is not a death sentence. Patients need to understand exactly what heart failure is, what might have caused it, why the symptoms occur and what the patient's prognosis might be. Good communication between the health care professional and the patient from this early stage are an essential part of empowering the patient to become involved in the management of their own disease.

Discussions with the patient and their relatives should then go on to cover such topics as how to recognize the worsening of symptoms and what to do if this occurs. In addition, this discussion should cover general lifestyle measures such as diet, the need for physical activity and the importance of weight management. Drug counselling is also vital: most patients will be on a number of drugs and compliance may be better when the patient (and their carer) are fully informed about the need for the different medications. The pharmacist will also be able to advise regarding medication.

LIFESTYLE MEASURES

Diet
Patients with heart failure should be encouraged to adopt lifestyle measures that are designed for ameliorating the sodium and fluid retention that is characteristic of the syndrome. The most important dietary adjustment that patients can make is to control their salt intake, which is

particularly important in those with advanced heart failure. Salt causes the body to retain fluid. In the Western world most of us take in too much salt, approximately 10 g per day. Reducing this by 50% in healthy patients will lead to a reduction in extracellular volume of 1.0–1.5 l and a reduction in weight of 1.0–1.5 kg.[1] What effect this will have in patients with heart failure is unknown, but excess quantities of salt certainly have the potential to counteract the effect of diuretics prescribed for reducing the symptoms of fluid retention.

Unfortunately a very low salt diet is unpalatable to most people. Patients may opt to use salt substitutes, although these should be used with caution as they may contain potassium. When used in large quantities, particularly in combination with an angiotensin-converting enzyme inhibitor, they may lead to hyperkalaemia.[2]

The simplest way that patients can reduce the amount of salt in their diet is to avoid adding salt to meals at the table, to cook with less salt (perhaps by using spices instead) and to avoid buying salted foods such as peanuts and snacks and products such as soy sauce. They should also be encouraged to avoid or at least to cut down on processed meats such as salami and ready-made convenience meals, as these tend to contain large quantities of salt.

Fluid retention is less severe in patients with mild heart failure, but those patients with advanced heart failure, with or without hyponatraemia, may also need to cut down their fluid intake to between 2.5 and 3.5 pints (1.5–2.0 l) each day (except in particularly hot weather). Many patients, particularly those who are elderly, tend to forget that drinks such as tea and coffee are mostly water.

Weight management and fluid balance
Patients should be encouraged to monitor their weight on a regular basis, ideally once or twice a week, in order to check on their fluid balance. If there is a sudden and

unexpected weight gain of more than 2 kg in 3 days they should contact a health care professional as their diuretics and/or other drugs may require dosage adjustments. However, many patients are able to manage their own diuretic dose adjustment within pre-agreed limits tailored to the individual patient. Several remote monitoring systems are being developed for assisting in the home monitoring of heart failure patients.

Smoking and alcohol

There are two 'social' habits that should be modified by patients with heart failure: smoking and alcohol.

Smoking is the major lifestyle risk factor for all forms of cardiovascular disease. Smoking is associated with significant haemodynamic effects in patients with heart failure that are potentially harmful, most notably an increase in myocardial oxygen consumption.[3]

Therefore, smoking should be discouraged at every possible opportunity. The use of smoking cessation programmes and appropriate aids for cessation such as nicotine replacement therapy should be actively encouraged.

All patients with heart failure should be advised to moderate their alcohol intake and those where alcoholic cardiomyopathy is suspected should be strongly advised to stop taking alcohol altogether. In these patients abstinence is associated with an improvement in their left ventricular ejection fraction and symptoms of heart failure.[4]

In patients in whom heart failure is not due to alcohol there is no evidence that light to moderate alcohol consumption impacts on prognosis.[5]

Erratic alcohol consumption may also affect the intensity of anticoagulation with warfarin and should be avoided in patients who require this medication.

Exercise and rest

Traditionally the advice for patients with chronic diseases such as heart failure has been to 'take it easy' and to take plenty of bed rest in the hope that this might minimize the symptoms.

Today the advice is that rest should *not* be encouraged in patients with stable chronic heart failure. In general, physical rest or bed rest is necessary only in cases of acute heart failure or when there is destabilization of chronic heart failure. In such cases passive mobilization exercise should be carried out in order to limit physical deconditioning and reduce the risks of venous thrombosis from prolonged bed rest. Respiratory exercises and active mobilization can then be initiated as the clinical condition of the patient improves.

Those patients living with stable heart failure should as far as is possible be encouraged to carry out daily physical activity, perhaps by continuing to work and to undertake leisure time activities, where these do not induce excessive symptoms, in order to prevent muscle deconditioning. As a rule, strenuous exercise and competitive sport should be discouraged.

Exercise training programmes

It is thought that the physiology of the muscle in heart failure undergoes a gradual metabolic change favouring catabolic over anabolic processes. This is thought to contribute to the muscle wasting seen in more severe disease. Evidence from a number of clinical studies suggests that exercise training programmes can help to prevent this dysfunction in skeletal muscle, thereby improving patients' functional capacity without causing any harm. One trial has even suggested that heart failure patients who undergo a 12-month programme experience significantly fewer adverse cardiac events compared with those who take no exercise.[6]

Various guidelines promote the use of exercise training programmes in stable patients with mild to moderate heart failure and standardized recommendations for exercise training in heart failure patients have been published by the European Society of Cardiology.[7]

Such programmes are associated with an increase in patients' physical capacity, while also improving the symptoms and patients' perceptions of their quality of life. Where available such programmes should be offered to those patients with stable heart failure who are most likely to benefit from them.

Sexual activity

There is a frequent association between sexual dysfunction and cardiovascular disease and sexual activity itself can pose a potential cardiac risk in patients with cardiovascular disease. Even though clinicians often find it difficult to discuss questions of sexual activity with patients and their partners it is clearly an issue that may have to be addressed. Simply counselling against any form of sexual activity is not appropriate, particularly as this can have an adverse effect on a patient's quality of life, well being and relationship with their partner.

Patients with mild (New York Heart Association class II) heart failure are thought to have an intermediate risk while those with moderate to severe (class III–IV) heart failure are at higher risk of decompensation triggered by sexual activity.[8,9]

Current recommendations are to provide reassurance for the not severely compromised but frightened patient and their partner (who may well be even more frightened) and perhaps to refer the couple for specialist counselling. Where appropriate advice might be given on the use of sublingual nitrates before sexual activity.

However, those at high risk should be referred for specialized cardiac evaluation and management and treatment for conditions such as erectile dysfunction should be deferred until the patient's cardiac condition has stabilized.

Travelling abroad

Many patients with heart failure worry about whether or not they are able to go on holiday or to travel abroad. In most cases there is no reason why they should not do so.

In general they should be discouraged from holidaying at high altitudes. Travelling to very hot or humid places is not advisable. Short air flights are preferable to long journeys by other forms of transport. In those with severe heart failure long air flights can cause problems, particularly with regard to dehydration, excessive limb oedema and deep venous thrombosis and patients should be warned about these risks. Patients should not be afraid to ask for help at the airport, particularly if they have to walk a long distance to the aeroplane.

Those travelling to hot humid climates may need to adapt their dosages of diuretics and other drugs in order to avoid losing too much sodium and fluid.

Vaccinations
Respiratory infections such as pneumococcal pneumonia and influenza may worsen heart failure. Patients should therefore be encouraged to obtain annual immunization against influenza every autumn, as well as a one-off immunization against pneumococcus.

Weight management
Patients with a body mass index (BMI) (i.e. actual weight in kilograms divided by height in metres squared) of between 25 and 30 kg/m^2 are classified as being overweight, while those with a BMI of >30 kg/m^2 are classified as obese. Being overweight or obese is associated with an increased risk of heart failure, usually mediated through obesity hypertension and the development of left ventricular hypertrophy.

Patients with chronic heart failure should be encouraged to lose weight if they are overweight or obese. Weight reduction in obese patients is associated with a reduction in symptoms such as breathlessness and fatigue. It is best achieved through a programme of calorie restriction and physical activity rather than by using currently available weight reducing drugs, some of which are contraindicated in patients with cardiovascular disease.

While excess weight is a problem in heart failure patients with mild disease, approximately 50% of patients with severe chronic heart failure show signs of clinical or subclinical malnutrition.[10]

Weight loss is common as heart disease progresses and may become extreme. Cardiac cachexia, the wasting of both fat and lean tissue that accompanies extreme weight loss, is an important predictor of reduced survival from heart failure.[11,12]

The general practitioner (GP) should consider the possibility of abnormal weight loss if a patient's body weight falls below 90% of their ideal body weight or if there is non-intentional weight loss of 5 kg or more than 7.5% of the previous normal body weight in the previous 6 months. Trials of various drugs including anabolic hormones and immune modulators are ongoing in

---

Case Study **Exercise training improved Joseph's outlook on life**

After he was diagnosed with heart failure, Joseph Brown felt rather downhearted about his situation. Initially, he felt he should take life as easily as possible. Since his wife did the shopping and housework he had little need to do much in the way of exercise.

However, he was urged by his GP to get out more, setting himself small achievable goals, such as walking to the letter box at the end of the road and then, when he was able to do that quite comfortably, to the paper shop in the High Street. The more he did, the more Joseph felt able to do.

Subsequently, the doctor suggested that he sign up for the exercise training programme at the local leisure centre. Although he was a bit nervous at first he agreed after a little encouragement from his wife. She said she would be glad to see him get out of the house twice a week!

At the leisure centre Joseph and the other cardiac patients were coached by professional trainers who assessed their exercise capacity by measuring their breathing and pulse rate in order to determine how much exercise they could safely take.

Each session then began with a warm-up phase of stretching exercises lasting for 10–15 min, followed by 30 min of exercise that involved jogging around the gym, cycling on the exercise bikes and doing some simple muscle strengthening exercises. Joseph's blood pressure and heart rate were measured at rest, before he started exercising, during the middle of exercising and again at the end of each session.

After some months of the sessions he realized that he felt much better about his heart disease and had a generally a more positive outlook on life. He also found that he could walk to the High Street with no difficulty – quite a change from only a short time before.

patients with cardiac cachexia, but in the meantime dietary supplementation would be sensible.

Family counselling

Coronary artery disease does of course have a genetic component. Patients with very high serum cholesterol levels may have a genetic hyperlipidaemia and this requires specialist assessment and screening within the first-degree relatives of the patient. However, several of the cardiomyopathies may also be genetic in origin. This applies particularly to hypertrophic cardiomyopathy, where an autosomal dominant gene defect may arise spontaneously or be passed from one generation to another. Screening for this condition in first-degree relatives of cases should be organized. This is usually done by echocardiography, but may be less than straightforward in first-degree relatives who are still children, as the condition may only become obvious as they get older. Specialist advice is strongly recommended. The Cardiomyopathy Association can provide support for such families and have a very informative World Wide Web site (http://www.cardiomyopathy.org).

REFERENCES

1. Antonios TF, MacGregor GA. Salt – more adverse effects. *Lancet* 1996; **348**: 250–1.
2. Good CB, McDermott L, McCloskey B. Diet and serum potassium in patients on ACE inhibitors. *JAMA* 1995; **274**: 538.
3. Nicolozakes AW, Binkley PF, Leier CV. Hemodynamic effects of smoking in congestive heart failure. *Am J Med Sci* 1988; **296**: 377–80.
4. Jacob AJ, McLaren KM, Boon NA. Effects of abstinence on alcoholic heart muscle disease. *Am J Cardiol* 1991; **68**: 805–7.
5. Cooper HA, Exner DV, Domanski MJ. Light-to-moderate alcohol consumption and prognosis in patients with left ventricular systolic dysfunction. *J Am Coll Cardiol* 2000; **35**: 1753–9.
6. Belardinelli R, Georgiou D, Cianci G, Purcaro A. Randomized, controlled trial of long-term moderate exercise training in chronic heart failure: effects on functional capacity, quality of life, and clinical outcome. *Circulation* 1999; **99**: 1173–82.
7. Working Group on Cardiac Rehabilitation and Exercise Physiology and Working Group on Heart Failure of the European Society of Cardiology. Recommendations for exercise testing in chronic heart failure patients. *Eur Heart J* 2001; **22**: 125–35.
8. DeBusk R, Drory Y, Goldstein I *et al*. Management of sexual dysfunction in patients with cardiovascular disease: recommendations of the Princeton Consensus Panel. *Am J Cardiol* 2000; **86**: 175–81.

9. Jackson G, Betteridge J, Dean J *et al*. A systematic approach to erectile dysfunction in the cardiovascular patient: a consensus statement. *Int J Clin Pract* 1999; **53**: 445–51.

10. McKee PA, Castelli WP, McNamara PM, Kannel WB. The natural history of congestive heart failure: the Framingham Study. *N Engl J Med* 1971; **285**: 1441–6.

11. Anker SD, Chua TP, Ponikowski P *et al*. Hormonal changes and catabolic/anabolic imbalance in chronic heart failure and their importance for cardiac cachexia. *Circulation* 1997; **96**: 526–34.

12. Anker SD, Ponikowski P, Varney S *et al*. Wasting as independent risk factor for mortality in chronic heart failure. *Lancet* 1997; **349**: 1050–3.

Chapter 4

Drug treatment of heart failure

Cardiac damage, whatever the cause, stimulates a large number of biochemical and physiological pathways. These may initially be compensatory, but in the longer term can be counterproductive.

Greater understanding of the body's response to cardiac damage has led to important advances in the pharmacological management of heart failure in recent years. As recently as 20 years ago the major treatment option was a diuretic ('water pills') combined with digoxin. Today, published guidelines for the treatment of heart failure[1] based on randomized, double-blind, placebo-controlled trials support the use of a growing range of drugs, enabling clinicians to tailor therapy in order to achieve the major aims of treatment. These include:

- relieving a patient's symptoms and improving the patient's quality of life
- preventing admission to hospital, recurrent ischaemic events and further deterioration in left ventricular function
- reducing mortality.

DIURETICS

Diuretics have not been shown to affect survival in patients with heart failure, but they do provide rapid relief from the symptoms and have formed the mainstay of therapy for several decades.[2] For patients with evidence of fluid retention, such as pulmonary congestion, raised jugular venous pressure, peripheral oedema or ascites, diuretics are of great benefit.

Treatment usually begins with a low dose of a diuretic, which may be increased until urine output increases, weight decreases and the tendency towards fluid retention is controlled.

Figure 4.1   The treatment algorithm for left ventricular dysfunction proposed in the National Service Framework for Coronary Heart Disease. (1) See the algorithm for the use of an ACE inhibitor in Fig. 4.2. If not tolerated, consider an angiotensin II receptor antagonist/H-ISDN combination therapy/digoxin. (2) Indicated in New York Heart Association (NYHA) class I–III heart failure. Extreme caution required in initiating beta blockers: this must be done under specialist care [see page 53/4 for more current advice on this group of drugs]. (3) Electrical cardioversion may be indicated and other specialist drugs such as amiodarone may be indicated. (4) Referral to a specialist with an interest in heart failure: coronary angiography and bypass surgery may be indicated. (5) Indicated in NYHA class III–IV heart failure. Dose of 25 mg once daily: extreme care must be taken to avoid hyperkalaemia and renal failure, i.e. monitor electrolytes carefully. (6) Other specialist therapy may be indicated as an outpatient or inpatient.

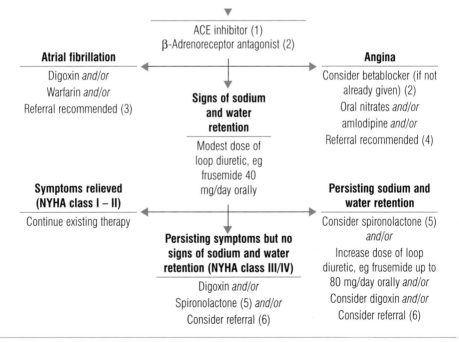

Treatment of left ventricular systolic dysfunction

Confirm diagnosis by echocardiography or radionuclide ventriculography. If possible discontinue aggravating drugs, e.g. non-steroid anti-inflammatory drugs (NSAIDs)
Address non-pharmacological and lifestyle measures

ACE inhibitor (1)
β-Adrenoreceptor antagonist (2)

Atrial fibrillation

Digoxin *and/or*
Warfarin *and/or*
Referral recommended (3)

Angina

Consider betablocker (if not already given) (2)
Oral nitrates *and/or*
amlodipine *and/or*
Referral recommended (4)

Signs of sodium and water retention

Modest dose of loop diuretic, eg frusemide 40 mg/day orally

Symptoms relieved (NYHA class I – II)

Continue existing therapy

Persisting sodium and water retention

Consider spironolactone (5) *and/or*
Increase dose of loop diuretic, eg frusemide up to 80 mg/day orally *and/or*
Consider digoxin *and/or*
Consider referral (6)

Persisting symptoms but no signs of sodium and water retention (NYHA class III/IV)

Digoxin *and/or*
Spironolactone (5) *and/or*
Consider referral (6)

In mild heart failure, thiazide diuretics may be used, whereas in moderate heart failure loop diuretics (such as frusemide, bumetanide or torasemide) are usually preferred.[3] For patients with more severe symptoms or resistant oedema thiazide diuretics and loop diuretics have a synergistic effect and may be used in combination for increasing diuresis, for example frusemide plus low dose metolazone. However, over-diuresis and electrolyte imbalances may occur and careful monitoring of renal function and potassium together with a regular review of doses are essential.

Once fluid retention has been controlled diuretic treatment is generally maintained at a level for preventing fluid build up, which may require frequent dose adjustment. Patients should be encouraged to record their weight each day; many may also be able to adjust their diuretic dose accordingly, although for those who cannot the general practitioner (GP) or a nurse should be available to provide assistance.

The timing of diuretics is flexible, so patients should be advised that morning doses can be delayed until later in the day when necessary, for example when the patient is travelling. Evening doses should be avoided because of inconvenient nocturia: if a second daily dose is required this is usually best in the early afternoon.

Diuretics are usually very effective at treating and controlling fluid retention, but they do not prevent disease progression. In fact, diuretic use appears to stimulate the renin–angiotensin–aldosterone system, which may therefore accelerate the disease process. This is why in cases of systolic dysfunction diuretics should not be used alone, even if the symptoms of heart failure are controlled, but combined wherever possible with an angiotensin-converting enzyme (ACE) inhibitor and a beta blocker (see below). In some patients after initial control of fluid retention the introduction of an ACE inhibitor and other treatment may permit the complete withdrawal of diuretics in due course.

Since most patients taking a diuretic will also be taking an ACE inhibitor, the use of potassium-sparing diuretics (such as triamterene or amiloride, combined with loop diuretics in several proprietary preparations) has traditionally been avoided due to the risk of hyperkalaemia. However, such combinations can be useful in patients who run a low potassium concentration and are to be preferred to potassium supplements. Spironolactone is a special case: its use in heart failure has enjoyed a resurgence recently as a result of a large clinical trial, but it is used in a very low dose with little effect on diuresis (or plasma potassium concentrations). This is discussed in more detail below.

NEUROHORMONAL ANTAGONISTS

ACE inhibitors

ACE inhibitors are the first choice of vasodilator agents and are indicated in all stages of symptomatic heart failure resulting from left ventricular systolic dysfunction (and also in patients with asymptomatic left ventricular systolic dysfunction).

ACE inhibitors appear to exert beneficial effects over and above vasodilatation, affecting processes such as ventricular remodelling and enlargement. These effects are mediated through blockade of the renin–angiotensin–aldosterone system. ACE inhibitors block the conversion of inactive angiotensin I to angiotensin II, which has vasoconstrictive, salt-retentive and cardiac hypertrophic properties. In addition, they cause the build up of bradykinin, which has vasodilatory and natriuretic properties. Bradykinin may also trigger a dry irritating cough, which may reduce patient adherence with treatment.

In a large range of randomized controlled clinical trials conducted in patients with heart failure due to left ventricular systolic dysfunction[4–10] ACE inhibitors have consistently been shown to:

- delay disease progression
- produce symptomatic relief

- produce improvements in functional capacity
- reduce the risk of hospitalization
- prolong survival.

Furthermore, ACE inhibitors have been shown to improve survival and decrease the risk of developing heart failure in patients who have had a recent myocardial infarction and have left ventricular systolic dysfunction with or without symptoms.[11-13] This cardioprotective effect was confirmed in high-risk patients in the Heart Outcomes Prevention Evaluation Study.[14]

However, despite this considerable body of evidence demonstrating efficacy and cost-effectiveness, ACE inhibitors are suboptimally prescribed in patients with heart failure. Recent studies assessing use among all patients with heart failure have suggested that only approximately one-half of patients discharged from hospital and one-quarter of community-dwelling patients were prescribed ACE inhibitors, with the doses used in practice often being substantially lower than those achieved in controlled trials.[15-17]

Higher doses of ACE inhibitors are associated with greater prognostic benefit than lower doses. The Assessment of Treatment with Lisinopril and Survival Study demonstrated a statistically significant 14% reduction in the relative risk of death and need for hospital admission during a period of 4 years, with a daily dosage of 32.5–35.0 mg lisinopril compared with 2.5–5 mg lisinopril.[18]

It is generally accepted that, where there are no contraindications, ACE inhibitors should be prescribed for the following.

1. All patients with left ventricular systolic dysfunction as evidenced by, for example, a low ejection fraction (<40–45%), whether or not they have symptoms of heart failure.

2. All patients who have suffered a myocardial infarction and have evidence of ventricular damage.

In general, ACE inhibitor side-effects are not dose related and effort must be made to get patients to the target doses used in clinical trials (see Table 4.1).

In practice it is important to advise patients that it may be several weeks before they notice an improvement in their symptoms. For those who achieve no symptomatic benefit and in whom compliance may be poor it should be explained that ACE inhibitors are helpful in reducing the progression of their disease.

Contraindications to the use of ACE inhibitors include renal artery stenosis, pregnancy, greatly increased plasma potassium concentrations or angio-oedema to previous exposure to ACE inhibitors. Hospital supervision is required for patients with low systolic blood pressure (<100 mmHg), the use of high-dose diuretics (frusemide 80 mg and above or equivalent each day) or a greatly increased serum creatinine concentration(>250 mmol/l). Regular monitoring of renal function is recommended before and 1–2 weeks after each dose increment and at 3 and 6 months. More frequent measurements may be

Table 4.1   Recommended doses of ACE inhibitors

Drug	Starting dose	Maintenance dose
Captopril	6.25 mg three times daily	25–50 mg three times daily
Cilazapril	0.5 mg once daily	1–2.5 mg once daily
Fosinopril	10 mg once daily	20 mg once daily
Enalapril	2.5 mg once daily	10 mg twice daily
Lisinopril	2.5 mg once daily	5–20 mg once daily
Quinapril	2.5–5 mg once daily	5–10 mg once daily
Perindopril	2 mg once daily	4 mg once daily
Ramipril	1.25–2.5 mg once daily	2.5–5 mg twice daily
Trandolapril	1 mg once daily	4 mg once daily

necessary in patients with a history of renal dysfunction or electrolyte disturbances (see Table 4.2).

Particular care needs to be paid to the initiation of ACE inhibitors. Historically, GPs have been reluctant to initiate ACE inhibitors. Concerns have centred on first-dose hypotension, particularly when large doses of earlier drugs such as captopril were used in patients with severe heart failure. Problems are rare in patients with mild or moderate heart failure who have normal renal function and a systolic blood pressure over 100 mmHg and who have stopped taking diuretics for at least 24 h. It is now accepted that most heart failure patients can safely be established on ACE inhibitors without the need for hospital admission. Nevertheless, it is sometimes prudent for the patient to take the first dose of their ACE inhibitor at night before going to bed. Table 4.2 provides some advice regarding the initiation of ACE inhibitors.

Table 4.2   Tips for the initiation of ACE inhibitors in heart failure patients in general practice

•   Measure blood pressure and determine electrolytes and creatinine concentrations before treatment is initiated
•   Consider referring 'high-risk' patients to hospital for assessment and supervision before treatment is started
•   Use ACE inhibitors with caution in patients with severe peripheral vascular disease because of the possible association with atherosclerotic renal artery stenosis (monitor serum creatinine particularly closely)
•   Increase doses gradually over 2–3 weeks, aiming for the target doses used in large clinical trials
•   Monitor blood pressure and electrolytes or renal chemistry once treatment has been started, initially at 1 week then less frequently: more frequent monitoring may be required if abnormalities are detected or if there is a higher risk of renal artery stenosis (e.g. patients with peripheral vascular disease)
•   NB: a small (<10%) increment in serum creatinine concentration on commencing therapy is not a reason for abandoning treatment; any greater rise should be discussed with a specialist

Confirmed left ventricular systolic ACE inhibitor

▼	▼

Specialist advice required before starting ACE inhibitor

If any of the following:

- Creatinine >200 μmol/l
- Urea >12mmol/l
- Sodium ≤ 130mmol/l
- Systolic arterial pressure <100 mm Hg
- Diuretic dose >frusemide 80 mg/day or equivalent
- Known or suspected renal artery stenosis, e.g. peripheral vascular disease

Suitable for treatment initiation in the community

Step 1

- Stop potassium supplement/potassium-sparing diuretic (because of risk of hyperkalaemia)
- If possible stop NSAID (because of risk of renal dysfunction)
- Before starting an ACE inhibitor, advise patient about possible symptomatic hypotension (i.e. dizziness, and lightheadedness)
- Start with low dose of an ACE inhibitor, e.g. enalapril 2.5 mg twice daily
- Titrate to an intermediate dose, e.g. enalapril 5 mg twice daily over first week

Step 2
Review patient after 1 week

Adverse effects ←

- Check blood chemistry (potassium, urea and creatinine)
- Check for adverse effects, e.g. symptomatic hypotension and renal dysfunction/hyperkalaemia (i.e. a rise in urea to ≥ 12 mmol/l, creatinine to ≥ 200μmol/l or potassium to ≥ 5.5 mmol/l)

No adverse effects

Specialist referral

- Aim for the target dose (or highest dose tolerated) of an ACE inhibitor (e.g. enalapril 10–20 mg twice daily) as these have been shown to reduce morbidity and mortality
- Titrate to this dose over a period of 1 month

Step 3
Review patient after 1 month

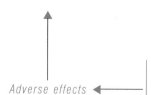

Adverse effects ←

- Check blood chemistry (potassium, urea and creatinine)
- Check for adverse effects, e.g. symptomatic hypotension and renal dysfunction/hyperkalaemia and intolerable cough

Angiotensin II receptor blockers

Angiotensin II is a highly potent vasoconstrictor. Whereas ACE inhibitors block its production, currently available angiotensin II receptor blockers (ARBs) block the action of angiotensin II predominantly at the type 1 receptor, leading to vasodilatation.

There are currently six ARBs available, with the following total daily doses.

1. Losartan 50–100 mg.

2. Valsartan 80–320 mg.

3. Candesartan cilexetil 4–16 mg.

4. Irbesartan 150–300 mg.

5. Telmisartan 40–80 mg.

6. Eprosartan 400–800 mg.

Although they are used primarily for the treatment of hypertension, ARBs demonstrated early promise in patients with heart failure and a number of these agents are currently under investigation in heart failure (see Table 4.3). As of 2002, none was licensed for the treatment of heart failure in the UK.

To date, ARBs have not been shown to be superior to ACE inhibitors, although they do appear to lack the bradykinin-related side-effect of ACE inhibitors and so they may be considered in patients who are unable to tolerate ACE inhibitors because of cough.[19,20] As with ACE inhibitors, monitoring of renal function remains essential.

It has been suggested that combining ACE inhibition with angiotensin receptor blockade may offer additional

Facing page

Figure 4.2   The Scottish Intercollegiate Guidelines Network algorithm for the use of ACE inhibitors (reproduced with permission from the Scottish Intercollegiate Guidelines Network. Diagnosis and Treatment of Heart Failure Due to Left Ventricular Systolic Dysfunction. Scottish Intercollegiate Guidelines Network Publication No 35; 1999).

benefits.[21] This strategy was studied in the ValHeFT trial, which showed a 13% reduction in combined mortality and morbidity, with a 27% reduction in hospitalization for worsening heart failure.[22] The ongoing CHARM study will provide further information on this combined strategy as it includes an arm in which patients with heart failure due to left ventricular dysfunction are randomized to placebo or candesartan in addition to an ACE inhibitor. In the meantime, the combination of an ARB with an ACE inhibitor should probably only be considered in patients who will not tolerate beta blockers

Table 4.3   Details of angiotensin II receptor antagonists used in clinical trials in heart failure

Drug	Trial
Losartan	Evaluation of Losartan in the Elderly II: losartan versus captopril in 3152 patients with NYHA class II–IV heart failure. Reported in 2000
	OPTIMAAL: losartan versus captopril in 5000 patients post-myocardial infarction with left ventricular dysfunction. Reported in 2002
Valsartan	ValHeFT: valsartan versus placebo in 5010 patients with NYHA class II–IV heart failure already on an ACE inhibitor (with or without a beta blocker). Although the primary end-point of mortality alone was similar in both groups, the combined mortality and morbidity end-point was reduced by 13% (relative risk), driven largely by a reduction in hospitalizations. Reported in 2002
	VALIANT: valsartan versus captopril versus valsartan plus captopril in 14 500 post-myocardial infarction patients with left ventricular dysfunction. Due to report in 2003
Candesartan	CHARM: a three-arm trial of candesartan in patients with a left ventricular ejection fraction <40% on an ACE inhibitor, candesartan in patients with a left ventricular ejection fraction <40% intolerant of ACE inhibitor and candesartan in patients with a left ventricular ejection fraction >40% ('diastolic heart failure'). Due to report in 2003
Irbesartan	I-PRESERVE: irbesartan versus placebo in 3600 patients over 60 years of age with symptomatic heart failure and a preserved systolic function (left ventricular ejection fraction >45%). Due to report in 2006

Beta blockers

Activation of the sympathetic nervous system is a contributory factor in the pathophysiology of heart failure. Initially this helps compensate for reduced pump function, but in the longer term this is harmful and results in structural changes that worsen heart failure and increase the risk of arrhythmia.

Traditionally beta blockers were thought to be contraindicated in patients with heart failure due to their acute negative inotropic effects. However, a large number of clinical trials have now provided evidence that beta blockade in addition to standard treatment with diuretics and ACE inhibitors prolongs survival, slows disease progression and reduces hospitalizations in patients with mild to severe heart failure due to left ventricular systolic dysfunction, irrespective of the underlying aetiology.[23-25]

However, it is essential that beta blockade is introduced at a very low dose and is increased in stages under appropriate supervision.

Three beta blockers, the β_1-adrenoceptor-selective metoprolol and bisoprolol and the non-selective β-adrenoceptor antagonist carvedilol, which also has alpha blocking properties, all have strong trial evidence to support their use in moderate (NYHA class II–III) heart failure. In addition, the recent Carvedilol Prospective Randomized Cumulative Survival Study has demonstrated the benefit of carvedilol in patients with severe heart failure.[26]

Consequently, unless contraindicated, all patients with mild to severe heart failure who have been stable for 2 months on diuretics and an ACE inhibitor should receive one of these beta blockers.

A 'start low and go slow' policy combined with adequate patient education should be adopted when commencing beta blockers as initially the patient's symptoms may worsen and it may take 2–3 months before an improvement is apparent, even though disease progression will be retarded even in the absence of symptomatic improvement.

Beta blocker dosages should be increased as side-effects resolve at lower doses.

Patients should be encouraged to monitor their weight daily after each dose increase and be advised on increasing their diuretic dose should a weight increase be seen. The dose should be increased to the target dose (see Table 4.4) or to the highest dose tolerated by the patient.

Traditionally the introduction and titration of beta blockade for patients with heart failure due to left ventricular systolic dysfunction has been the province of hospital doctors. However, this process is increasingly being performed in primary care. Experience in monitoring such patients and adjusting heart failure therapy is advisable.

Spironolactone

As well as reducing circulating levels of angiotensin, ACE inhibitors and angiotensin II receptor antagonists also reduce circulating levels of aldosterone, albeit to varying degrees.

Table 4.4   Starting dose, target dose and titration scheme for beta blockers

Beta blocker	First dose	Increments	Target dose	Titration period
Carvedilol	3.125 mg twice daily	6.25, 12.5, 25 and 50	25 mg twice daily	Weeks–month
Bisoprolol	1.25 mg once daily	2.5, 3.75, 5, 7.5 and 10	10 mg once daily	Weeks–month
Metoprolol tartrate	5 mg three times daily	10, 15, 30, 50, 75 and 100	50 mg three times daily	Weeks–month
Metoprolol succinate CR	12.5/25 mg once daily	25, 50, 100 and 200	200 mg once daily	Weeks–month

This table is based on data from large randomized clinical trials. Not all agents and dosages may be available or licensed.

Aldosterone plays an important role in the pathophysiology of heart failure by promoting adverse effects on cardiac structure and function, notably vascular and myocardial fibrosis, potassium and magnesium depletion, sodium retention, sympathetic activation, parasympathetic inhibition and baroreceptor dysfunction.

The aldosterone antagonist spironolactone was initially used as a potassium-sparing diuretic. However, at low doses it has been shown to have a mortality benefit in patients with severe heart failure. In the Randomized Aldactone Evaluation Study (RALES), spironolactone (12.5–50 mg) added to an ACE inhibitor and a loop diuretic improved survival in patients in severe heart failure (NYHA class III and IV), irrespective of aetiology.[27] Whether or not aldosterone antagonism has the same effect on reducing mortality and hospitalization in patients with mild heart failure (NYHA class II) or asymptomatic left ventricular dysfunction has yet to be established.

Adding a potassium-sparing diuretic to a patient who is already receiving an ACE inhibitor raises concerns of hyperkalaemia, particularly in patients who are elderly, diabetic or have renal dysfunction. Therefore, careful monitoring of patients' serum biochemistry is essential: serum potassium should be maintained <5.0 mmol/l and creatinine <250 mmol/l. Spironolactone should be added at 25 mg daily, with serum potassium and creatinine checked again after 4–6 days.

Unfortunately, however, spironolactone also affects oestrogen and androgen receptors; in the RALES trial 10% of patients developed gynaecomastia. These side-effects may be less of an issue with the new selective aldosterone receptor antagonist eplerenone, which is currently being studied in the Eplerenone Post-AMI for Heart Failure Efficacy and Survival Study.[28]

Digoxin
Cardiac glycosides such as digoxin are indicated in patients with heart failure and associated atrial fibrillation for controlling the ventricular rate and improving

ventricular function and symptoms. However, its use in patients with mild to moderate heart failure and sinus rhythm is less clear, despite studies addressing this issue.

In the Prospective Randomized Study of Ventricular Failure and Efficacy of Digoxin and the Randomized Assessment of Effect of Digoxin on Inhibitors of ACE Study[29,30] placebo was substituted in patients previously stabilized on digoxin. Both showed that there was a general worsening of heart failure, with fewer hospitalizations occurring in those patients who remained on digoxin.

The Digoxin Investigation Group Study assessed the effect of digoxin on morbidity and mortality when added to standard therapy of a diuretic and an ACE inhibitor.[31] It found that digoxin had no significant effect on overall mortality, although hospitalizations due to heart failure were decreased compared with placebo. Treatment with digoxin resulted in fewer deaths from the progression of heart failure, but there was an increase in other cardiac deaths, including arrhythmias.

The use of digoxin in patients with heart failure due to left ventricular systolic dysfunction taking the modern combination of diuretics, ACE inhibitors and beta blockers (and, in severe heart failure, also spironolactone) has not been assessed. In the UK digoxin is used less than in other parts of Europe or North America, generally being used for patients with heart failure and atrial fibrillation or patients with heart failure due to left ventricular systolic dysfunction who remain symptomatic despite optimal therapy with a diuretic, ACE inhibitor and beta blocker.

The usual daily oral dose of digoxin is 0.25–0.375 mg if serum creatinine is in the normal range. Due to decreased renal excretion in the elderly, a dose of 0.0625–0.125 mg is recommended. No loading dose is required when treating chronic conditions. Serum creatinine and potassium should be measured before initiating this drug, as hypokalaemia or hyperkalaemia increase the risk of arrhythmia with digoxin. Patients with renal dysfunction will require a reduction in dosage and advice should be sought.

Amiodarone and other anti-arrhythmic agents

Most anti-arrhythmic agents are best avoided in patients with heart failure, the only exceptions being beta blockers, which have been shown to reduce mortality, including sudden death, in heart failure (see the earlier section on neurohormonal antagonists) and the class III anti-arrhythmic amiodarone.

Amiodarone may be an effective agent for restoring sinus rhythm in heart failure patients with co-existing atrial fibrillation. However, its place in the treatment of heart failure patients is controversial. In the Grupo de Estudio de la Sobrevida en la Insuficiencia Cardiaca en Argentina Study low-dose amiodarone reduced mortality and hospital admission in patients with severe heart failure independently of the presence of complex ventricular arrhythmias. However, this result was not confirmed in the Survival Trial of Antiarrhythmic Therapy in Congestive Heart Failure in which prophylactic amiodarone suppressed ventricular arrhythmias and improved ventricular function, but did not reduce the incidence of sudden death or prolong survival among patients with congestive heart failure and asymptomatic ventricular arrhythmia.[33,34] In general, amiodarone is only recommended for patients who have symptomatic ventricular arrhythmias. Internal cardiac defibrillators are increasingly being used in preference to relying only on amiodarone in such patients (see Chapter 5).

Treatment with amiodarone is associated with side-effects, including hypothyroidism and hyperthyroidism, photosensitivity, conduction disturbances and bradycardia and, more rarely, pulmonary fibrosis, hepatic dysfunction and neuropathy. Corneal micro-deposits occur, but rarely cause symptoms and regress on stopping treatment. It is recommended that patients should have a chest X-ray and blood tests for thyroid and liver function before treatment and a check on thyroid and liver function 6 monthly thereafter. Any change in breathlessness in such patients will require further, more specialist assessment: pulmonary fibrosis is rare and it is more likely that changes in breathlessness will reflect changes in the control of the heart failure syndrome.

The decision to initiate and continue therapy with amiodarone should be taken by a physician experienced in the management of heart failure and arrhythmias. In most cases this will be a hospital specialist. If the indication for amiodarone therapy no longer holds then the prescription should be reviewed.

Other vasodilator agents
Hydralazine and isosorbide dinitrate
Vasodilator agents such as a combination of oral hydralazine and isosorbide dinitrate may be used as an adjunctive therapy in the management of heart failure in patients with concomitant angina or for the relief of acute dyspnoea. In addition, the combination has been advocated for patients in whom ACE inhibitors are contraindicated or are not tolerated because of cough. In the latter situation, ARBs are increasingly preferred.

When used in high doses, hydralazine and isosorbide dinitrate have been shown to improve survival in patients with heart failure compared with placebo, although the effect was inferior to enalapril; there was no beneficial effect on hospitalizations.

Alpha blockers
There is at present no evidence to support the use of a-adrenergic blockers in heart failure.

Calcium channel blockers
The use of rate-limiting calcium channel blockers such as diltiazem and verapamil is not recommended for patients with heart failure due to systolic dysfunction as they may further impair ventricular pump function and worsen heart failure. Newer long-acting agents of the

dihydropyridine class, such as amlopidine and felodipine, have shown no impact on survival in heart failure, but may be used as an additional therapy for patients with angina or concomitant hypertension. The ankle swelling that may occur with these agents may confuse the clinical picture and make assessment of the control of the heart failure syndrome more difficult.

Anti-thrombotic and anti-platelet agents

Oral anticoagulants (such as warfarin) have been shown to reduce the risk of death or thromboembolic events among patients with heart failure and co-existing atrial fibrillation. However, at present there is little evidence to indicate whether the long-term effect of anticoagulant or anti-platelet therapy contributes to mortality reduction in patients with left ventricular dysfunction who are in sinus rhythm rather than atrial fibrillation. Large-scale, prospective, randomized, controlled trials of anti-thrombotic therapies in patients with heart failure are in progress. The Warfarin and Antiplatelet Therapy in Chronic Heart Failure Study for instance is comparing the efficacy of aspirin, clopidogrel and warfarin and will provide much needed information. Interestingly, this study does not have a placebo arm, suggesting a consensus among clinicians that patients with heart failure should be on some form of anti-platelet or anticoagulant therapy until further data emerge.

Current recommendations suggest that anti-thrombotic or anti-platelet therapy is appropriate for patients with heart failure in several situations.

- Those patients with atrial fibrillation, in whom anticoagulation is essential unless the risk of haemorrhage is considered unacceptable. Anti-platelet agents are likely to be less effective in reducing the risk of thromboembolism, but would be preferred to no anti-thrombotic therapy.

- Those patients with a previous thromboembolism in whom anticoagulation is strongly recommended (or anti-platelet therapy if anticoagulation is not considered acceptable).

• Those patients with a history of coronary artery disease, in whom secondary prophylaxis with aspirin (or an oral anticoagulant) is generally recommended.

• Those patients with intracardiac thrombus, particularly if the thrombus is mobile and not layered, in whom anticoagulation is generally recommended.

• In some patients the relative risks and benefits of oral anticoagulation are finely balanced. Discussion with a hospital specialist may help.

Inotropic agents

Digoxin has inotropic action and has been discussed earlier in this chapter. Other inotropic agents are used intravenously in hospitalized patients with acutely decompensated heart failure. The most commonly used inotrope is the β-adrenoceptor agonist dobutamine. However, it is associated with tachycardia and increases the risk of serious arrhythmias. Milrinone is a phosphodiesterase inhibitor that also acts to increase cyclic adenosine 3'-5'-phosphate (cAMP) concentrations in the cardiac muscle cells. Despite its beneficial haemodynamic actions, in the Prospective Randomized Milrinone Survival Evaluation long-term therapy with the oral preparation of milrinone increased both the morbidity and mortality of patients with severe chronic heart failure.[35]

Occasionally patients become dependent on intravenous inotropic therapy and may be discharged home on this treatment under close supervision of the heart failure team.

Newer inotropic agents such as the calcium-sensitizing agent levosimendan increase the sensitivity of the contractile apparatus to calcium without increasing intracellular cAMP or calcium. Trials suggest that levosimendan results in an improvement in symptoms and haemodynamics.[36] Its place in the treatment of acute decompensated heart failure is not yet clear.

Investigational therapies
Despite the availability of the agents listed above, mortality from heart failure remains high. A number of other mechanisms involved in the pathogenesis of heart failure are now providing useful targets for future drug development. There are a large number of clinical trials currently recruiting patients, but the results of these are unlikely to influence the management of heart failure for some years.

Endothelin antagonism
The endothelins are a family of three powerfully vasoconstrictive neurohormones produced by the endothelium that play a role in maintaining cardiovascular homeostasis. Endothelin concentrations are elevated in chronic heart failure and parallel the symptomatic and haemodynamic severity of the syndrome. Therefore, both endothelin receptor antagonism and inhibition of endothelin-converting enzyme represent potential pharmacological targets.

However, the Research on Endothelin Antagonism in Chronic Heart Failure Study found that initiation of bosentan therapy was associated with an increased risk of worsening heart failure, although long-term therapy with bosentan may have improved the symptoms and favourably altered the progression of heart failure.

The effect of low-dose bosentan on mortality and morbidity in patients with severe heart failure was studied in the Endothelin Antagonist Bosentan for Lowering Cardiac Events in Heart Failure Study. Preliminary results have been presented showing that treatment with bosentan conferred an early risk of worsening heart failure, necessitating hospitalization as a consequence of fluid retention. The result has cast doubt on the potential benefits of non-specific endothelin receptor blockade in heart failure.

Endothelin-converting enzyme inhibitors have been less studied to date, although they are thought to have some therapeutic potential in chronic heart failure when combined with a neutral endopeptidase inhibitor, thus also raising circulating concentrations of natriuretic peptides.

Vasopeptidase inhibitors

Vasopeptidase inhibitors inhibit both ACE and neutral endopeptidase, the enzymatic pathway by which natriuretic peptides and kinins are degraded. The effect of stimulating the natriuretic peptide and kinin systems is to reduce vasoconstriction and enhance vasodilatation and diuresis.

The first vasopeptidase inhibitor studied in humans was omapatrilat. In patients with mild to moderate heart failure, omapatrilat was associated with improvements in functional class, but there was a higher incidence of angio-oedema than found with ACE inhibitors. Mortality trials are currently under way with omapatrilat. However, the Omapatrilat Versus Enalapril Randomized Trial of Utility in Reducing Events found no significant difference in mortality between the omapatrilat and enalapril groups.

Cytokine antagonists

Levels of various cytokines such as tumour necrosis factor-α (TNF-α) have been shown to be elevated in several disease states characterized by weight loss and cachexia, including severe heart failure. These cytokines are associated with depressed myocardial contractility, myocyte death and worsened prognosis.[37,38]

Studies involving non-specific TNF-a suppression using agents such as pentoxifylline have suggested an improvement in symptoms and left ventricular systolic function in patients with idiopathic dilated cardio-myopathy.[39]

In patients with advanced heart failure, treatment with the recombinant human TNF-α receptor blocker etanercept for 3 months was safe and well-tolerated and

resulted in a dose-dependent improvement in the left
ventricular ejection fraction and left ventricular
remodelling and a trend towards improvement in
functional status.[40]

However, larger and longer etanercept trials have been
terminated early through lack of efficacy. A trial using the
TNF-α monoclonal antibody infliximab was stopped
prematurely because of increased rates of mortality and
hospitalization in the active treatment group.

TREATMENT OF HEART FAILURE DUE TO DIASTOLIC DYSFUNCTION OF THE LEFT VENTRICLE

A substantial minority of patients with heart failure have
no abnormality of systolic function of the left ventricle
and no significant valve disease, but proven or presumed
'diastolic dysfunction' of the left ventricle. This is
particularly the case for very elderly patients and those
with a history of poorly controlled hypertension. The
evidence base for the treatment of such cases is not nearly
as large as that for heart failure due to systolic dysfunction
of the left ventricle. Most specialists would use a
combination of low- to moderate-dose diuretic therapy
with ACE inhibition (or an ARB if the patient cannot
tolerate an ACE inhibitor because of cough). Beta
blockade can also be used in an attempt to improve
relaxation of the left ventricle and, in carefully selected
situations, a calcium antagonist such as verapamil may be
recommended. Specialist advice is likely to be of benefit in
patients who do not respond to therapy with a diuretic
and ACE inhibitor.

TREATMENT OF HEART FAILURE DUE TO VALVE DISEASE

If the primary aetiology of the heart failure is valve
disease, then diuretic therapy is likely to be safe. ACE
inhibition and other vasodilator therapy should be
avoided in patients with more than mild aortic or mitral

valve stenosis, although this therapy can be very useful in patients with aortic or mitral valve regurgitation. Assessment regarding the need for surgical intervention is vital and a specialist centre will follow up most patients with valve disease.

TREATMENT OF OTHER CAUSES OF HEART FAILURE

Other rarer causes of heart failure (see Table 1.1 on page 6) will likely require specialist advice regarding management and are likely to be followed up closely by the specialist centre.

DRUG COUNSELLING

Compliance with drug treatments is crucial if patients are to gain the benefits of treatment, but is notoriously poor among all patients with chronic diseases. In the case of heart failure, poor adherence to medication is associated with the risk of deterioration and rehospitalization.

It is important to explain to patients the rationale for any drug treatments given and the effects that can be expected. This should stress that improvement in symptoms may be gradual and only complete after several weeks or even months with some drugs. Patients need to understand and accept that there is a need for gradual titration to the correct dosage levels with some drugs and that there may be no symptomatic relief and, furthermore, that this will require continued attendance at the clinic.

Patients should be given details of all drug dosages and suggestions for the time of administration and details of what to do in case of skipped doses.

In addition, any potential side-effects and adverse effects should be explained to the patient, particularly the risk of a dry cough and a decrease in taste with ACE inhibitors. They should be told that if dehydration occurs, for example as a result of diarrhoea or profuse sweating (particularly in hot climates), they should reduce the dose of their diuretics. Similarly, they should reduce the diuretic and, if necessary, temporarily reduce the ACE inhibitor dose if they experience symptomatic hypotension.

Importantly, this element of drug counselling should also focus on the range of drugs that patients should be encouraged to avoid taking.

Drugs that should be avoided or used with care by patients with chronic heart failure

There are a number of drugs that should be avoided or used with caution when co-prescribed with any form of heart failure treatment. The major drugs that GPs should be aware of are the following.

- **NSAIDs,** including over-the-counter drugs such as ibuprofen and the newer prescription-only cyclo-oxygenase-2-specific drugs, may worsen or precipitate heart failure, particularly in the elderly. In addition, they lessen the effectiveness of diuretics and may cause renal dysfunction and hyperkalaemia in patients taking potassium-sparing diuretics and ACE inhibitors

- **Class I anti-arrhythmics,** such as quinidine and flecainide, which have pro-arrhythmic effects on the ventricle and an adverse effect on haemodynamics and prognosis in heart failure

- **Calcium channel blockers,** particularly the rate-limiting non-dihydropyridines verapamil and diltiazem and the first-generation dihydropyridine derivatives such as nifedipine, may worsen ventricular function. Amlodipine and felodipine appear to be safe, but may cause ankle swelling

- **Tricyclic antidepressants,** such as imipramine, amitriptyline, clomipramine, dothiepin, lofepramine or nortriptyline, may increase the risk of arrhythmia. Newer generation antidepressants such as the selective serotonin reuptake inhibitors may be safer, but can still cause problems with hypotension and arrhythmia

- **Parenteral corticosteroids** such as prednisolone increase fluid retention.

- **Lithium** easily reaches toxic levels in patients on diuretics due to reduced excretion.

- **St John's wort** (*Hypericum perforatum*) is commonly bought over the counter as a natural remedy for depression. It may decrease the circulating levels and action of drugs such as warfarin and digoxin and should be avoided in patients taking these drugs. Importantly, different preparations of St John's wort may have different doses of the active ingredients and switching from one preparation to another may also influence blood levels of digoxin and warfarin.

Many patients with heart failure will be taking oral anticoagulants such as warfarin. Close attention to anticoagulant control is essential, particularly when changes are made in other medications, for example antibiotics or amiodarone. Patients should be warned to avoid taking additional aspirin and other NSAIDs as this increases the risk of bleeding. Many over-the-counter flu and cold remedies contain these compounds and patients should be encouraged always to ask the pharmacist's advice before purchasing drugs in the chemist.

IN SUMMARY

The modern pharmacological management of heart failure is based on polypharmacy. Many treatments have been proven to prolong survival and improve symptoms in large, well-conducted clinical trials. This evidence base has been enshrined in well-respected national and international clinical guidelines.[1]

Yet despite the availability of these treatments, mortality from heart failure remains high. While current investigation is focusing on other pathophysiological mechanisms and the interruption of these pathways, surveys consistently show that the use of currently available interventions such as ACE inhibitors and beta blockers is suboptimal, both in primary and secondary care. This indicates a need for greater efforts to increase both dosages and rates of prescribing of these agents.

Patient self-management is an important part of the treatment of heart failure and patients need to understand and use their medication in the most beneficial manner. Methods of facilitating this are discussed further in Chapter 6.

REFERENCES

1. The Task Force for the Diagnosis and Treatment of Chronic Heart Failure, European Society of Cardiology. Guidelines for the diagnosis and treatment of chronic heart failure. *Eur Heart J* 2001; **22**: 1527–60.
2. Faris R, Flather M, Purcell H *et al*. Current evidence supporting the role of diuretics in heart failure: a meta analysis of randomised controlled trials. *Int J Cardiol* 2002; **82**: 149–58.
3. Cosin J, Diez J on behalf of the Torasemide in Chronic Heart Failure Investigators. Torasemide in chronic heart failure: results of the TORIC Study. *Eur J Heart Failure* 2002; **4**: 507–13.
4. The SOLVD Investigators. Effect of enalapril on patients with reduced left ventricular ejection fractions and congestive heart failure. *N Engl J Med* 1991; **325**: 293–302.
5. The Cooperative North Scandinavian Enalapril Survival Study Trial Study Group. Effect of enalapril on mortality in severe congestive heart failure: results of the Cooperative North Scandinavian Enalapril Survival Study (CONSENSUS). *N Engl J Med* 1987; **316**: 1429–53.
6. Cohn JN, Johnson G, Zuesche S *et al*. A comparison of enalapril with hydralazine–isosorbide dinitrate in the treatment of chronic congestive heart failure. *N Engl J Med* 1991; **325**: 303–10.
7. The Captopril–Digoxin Multicenter Research Group. Comparative effects of therapy with captopril and digoxin in patients with mild to moderate heart failure. *JAMA* 1988; **259**: 539–44.
8. Garg R, Yusef S for the Collaborative Group on ACE-inhibitor Trials. Overview of randomized trials of angiotensin-converting enzyme inhibitors on mortality and morbidity in patients with heart failure. *JAMA* 1995; **273**: 1450–6.
9. Vantrimpont P, Rouleau JL, Wun CC *et al*. Additive beneficial effects of beta-blockers to angiotensin-converting enzyme inhibitors in the Survival and Ventricular Enlargement (SAVE) Study. SAVE Investigators. *J Am Coll Cardiol* 1997; **29**: 229–36.
10. Acute Infarction Ramipril Efficacy Study Investigators. Effect of ramipril on mortality and morbidity of survivors of acute myocardial infarction with clinical evidence of heart failure. *Lancet* 1993; **342**: 821–8.
11. Pfeffer MA, Braunwald E, Moy LA *et al* on behalf of the Survival and Ventricular Enlargement Investigators. Effect of captopril on mortality and morbidity in patients with left ventricular dysfunction after myocardial infarction: results of the Survival and Ventricular Enlargement Trial. *N Engl J Med* 1992; **327**: 669–77.
12. Kober L, Torp-Pederson C, Carlson JE *et al*. for the Trandolapril Cardiac Event Study Group. A clinical trial of the angiotensin-converting enzyme inhibitor trandolapril in patients with left ventricular dysfunction after myocardial infarction *N Engl J Med* 1995; **333**: 1670–6.
13. The SOLVD Investigators. Effect of enalapril on mortality and the development of heart failure in asymptomatic patients with reduced left ventricular ejection fractions. *N Engl J Med* 1992; **327**: 685–91.

14. The Heart Outcomes Prevention Evaluation Study Investigators. The effects of an angiotensin-converting enzyme inhibitor ramipril, on cardiovascular events in high risk patients. *N Engl J Med* 2000; **342**: 145–53.

15. Hobbs FDR. Management of heart failure: evidence versus practice. Does current prescribing provide optimal treatment for heart failure patients? *Br J Gen Pract* 2000; **50**: 735–42.

16. Bungard TJ, McAlister FA, Johnson JA, Tsuyaki RT. Under-utilisation of ACE-inhibitors in patients with congestive heart failure. *Drugs* 2001; **61**(14): 2021–33.

17. Hobbs FD, Jones MI, Allan TF *et al.* European survey of primary care physician perceptions on heart failure diagnosis and management (Euro-HF). *Eur Heart J* 2000; **21**: 1877–87.

18. Packer M, Poole-Wilson PA, Armstrong PW *et al.* Comparative effects of low doses and high doses of the angiotensin converting enzyme inhibitor, lisinopril, on morbidity and mortality in chronic heart failure. *Circulation* 1999; **100**: 2312–18.

19. Pitt B, Segal R, Martinez FA *et al.* on behalf of the Evaluation of Losartan in the Elderly Study Investigators. Randomised trial of losartan versus captopril in patients over 65 with heart failure (Evaluation of Losartan in the Elderly Study, ELITE). *Lancet* 1997; **349**: 747–52.

20. Pitt B, Poole-Wilson P, Segal R *et al.* on behalf of the Evaluation of Losartan in the Elderly Study Investigators. Effect of losartan versus captopril on mortality in patients with symptomatic heart failure: randomised trial – the Losartan Heart Failure Survival Study ELITE II. *Lancet* 2000; **355**: 1582–7.

21. Cohn JN, Tognoni G. A randomized trial of the angiotensin-receptor blocker valsartan in chronic heart failure. *N Engl J Med* 2001; **345**: 1667–75.

22. McKelvie RS, Yusuf S, Pericak D *et al.* Comparison of candesartan, enalapril, and their combination in congestive heart failure: Randomized Evaluation of Strategies for Left Ventricular Dysfunction (RESOLVD) Pilot Study. The RESOLVD Pilot Study Investigators. *Circulation* 1999; **100**: 1056–64.

23. Packer M, Bristow M, Cohn J *et al.* for the US Carvedilol Heart Failure Study Group. The effects of carvedilol on morbidity and mortality in patients with chronic heart failure. *N Engl J Med* 1996; **334**: 1349–55.

24. Cardiac Insufficiency Bisoprolol Study II Investigators. The Cardiac Insufficiency Bisoprolol Study II (CIBIS-II): a randomised trial. *Lancet* 1999; **353**: 9–13.

25. Metoprolol CR/XL Randomised Intervention Trial in Congestive Heart Failure Study Group. Effect of metoprolol CR/XL in chronic heart failure: Metoprolol CR/XL Randomised Intervention Trial in Congestive Heart Failure. *Lancet* 1999; **353**: 2001–7.

26. Packer M, Coats AJS, Fowler MB *et al.* for the Carvedilol Prospective Randomized Cumulative Survival Study Group. Effect of carvedilol on survival in severe chronic heart failure. *N Engl J Med* 2001; **344**: 1651–8.

27. Pitt B, Zannad F, Remme WJ *et al.* The effect of spironolactone on morbidity and mortality in patients with severe heart failure. *N Engl J Med* 1999; **341**: 709–17.

28. Pitt B, Williams G, Remme W *et al.* The EPHESUS Trial: eplerenone in patients with heart failure due to systolic dysfunction complicating acute myocardial infarction. Eplerenone Post-AMI Heart Failure Efficacy and Survival Study. *Cardiovasc Drugs Ther* 2001; **15**: 79–87.

29. Uretsky BF, Young JB, Shalidi FE *et al.* Randomised study assessing the effect of digoxin withdrawal in patients with mild to moderate chronic

heart failure: results of the PROVED Trial. *J Am Coll Cardiol* 1993; **22**: 955–62.

30. Packer M, Gheorghiade M, Young JB *et al.* Withdrawal of digoxin from patients with chronic heart failure treated with angiotensin-converting-enzyme inhibitors. RADIANCE Study. *N Engl J Med* 1993; **329**: 1–7.

31. The Digitalis Investigation Group. The effect of digoxin on mortality and morbidity in patients with heart failure. *N Engl J Med* 1997; **336**: 525–33.

32. Doval HC, Nul DR, Grancelli HO *et al.* Randomised trial of low-dose amiodarone in severe congestive heart failure. Grupo de Estudio de la Sobrevida en la Insuficiencia Cardiaca en Argentina (GESICA). *Lancet* 1994; **344**: 493–8.

33. Singh SN, Fletcher RD, Fisher SG *et al.* Amiodarone in patients with congestive heart failure and asymptomatic ventricular arrhythmia. Survival Trial of Antiarrhythmic Therapy in Congestive Heart Failure. *N Engl J Med* 1995; **333**: 77–82.

34. Massie BM, Fisher SG, Radford M *et al.* Effect of amiodarone on clinical status and left ventricular function in patients with congestive heart failure. CHF-STAT Investigators. *Circulation* 1996; **93**: 2128–34.

35. Packer M, Carver JR, Rodeheffer RJ *et al.* Effect of oral milrinone on mortality in severe chronic heart failure. The PROMISE Study Research Group. *N Engl J Med* 1991; **325**: 1468–75.

36. Slawsky MT, Colucci WS, Gottlieb SS *et al.* Acute hemodynamic and clinical effects of levosimendan in patients with severe heart failure. *Circulation* 2000; **102**: 2222–7.

37. Seta Y, Shan K, Bozkurt B, Oral H, Mann DL. Basic mechanisms in heart failure: the cytokine hypothesis. *J Card Failure* 1996; **2**: 243–9.

38. Levine B, Kalman J, Mayer L *et al.* Elevated circulating levels of tumor necrosis factor in severe chronic heart failure. *N Engl J Med* 1990; **323**: 236–41.

39. Sliwa K, Skudicky D, Candy G *et al.* Randomised investigation of effects of pentoxifylline on left ventricular performance in idiopathic dilated cardiomyopathy. *Lancet* 1998; **351**: 1091–3.

40. Bozkurt B, Torre-Amione G, Warren MS *et al.* Results of targeted anti-tumor necrosis factor therapy with etanercept (ENBREL) in patients with advanced heart failure. *Circulation* 2001; **103**: 1044–7.

Chapter 5

Surgery and other invasive interventions

Diagnostic investigations may identify a distinct under-lying cardiac abnormality that can be corrected by surgery or some other non-pharmacological intervention. There are three main situations in which non-pharmacological interventions may be advisable.

1. Where the patient's heart failure is due to coronary heart disease. In this situation revascularization by either percutaneous transluminal coronary angioplasty or by coronary artery bypass surgery may be advisable. This is currently the case for patients with co-existing angina that is not responding to medical treatment. However, there is growing evidence that some patients with no angina but a substantial amount of hibernating myocardium (heart muscle that is alive but not contracting) may benefit from coronary artery bypass surgery. The results of further trials are awaited.

2. Where the patient's heart failure is due to a damaged heart valve.

3. Where the patient's heart failure is severe and is not being controlled by drug treatments. In this situation, referral for heart transplantation may be advisable provided the patient is psychologically and physically fit enough to cope with the rigours of undergoing a major operation. Close follow-up post-operatively and immunosuppressive therapy is then needed. However, given the limited number of donor hearts available, this is only likely to be an option for a very small number of patients. If a donor heart is not immediately available and the patient is critically ill, then temporary support with a left ventricular assist device may be available in some centres.

Each of these options first requires the patient to undergo a specialist assessment by a cardiologist or cardiac surgeon.

REVASCULARIZATION

Coronary revascularization procedures are usually offered to patients with heart failure of ischaemic origin who experience the symptoms of angina. Revascularization can relieve the symptoms of ischaemia[1,2] and coronary artery bypass grafting surgery has been shown to reduce angina and reduce the risk of death in patients with multivessel coronary artery disease, systolic dysfunction and stable angina.[3,4]

Candidates for revascularization may need a considerable amount of counselling before their operation. The nature of the procedure, its risks and implications regarding time in hospital and the subsequent recovery time should be carefully explained to the patient. Following a bypass operation, patients should be offered the opportunity of taking part in a cardiac rehabilitation programme that includes regular exercise sessions and advice on healthy eating and relaxation techniques.

VALVE REPAIR/REPLACEMENT

Provided the operative risk is acceptable, patients with heart failure due to severe mitral valve insufficiency and those with secondary mitral insufficiency due to stretching of the mitral valve annulus due to left ventricular dilatation may obtain symptomatic improvement from mitral valve surgery or repair. Mitral stenosis is now relatively uncommon in the Western world, but heart failure due to this can be treated by mitral valvuloplasty (either by a surgeon or by a cardiologist using balloon valvuloplasty). Similarly, heart failure due to aortic valve disease can be treated by aortic valve replacement, provided the left ventricle is still functioning reasonably well.

Patients will need to be counselled regarding the nature of the procedure, its risks and implications regarding time in hospital and the subsequent recovery time.

Following a valve operation, patients should be offered the opportunity of taking part in a cardiac rehabilitation programme.

In situations where a new valve is fitted, patients will need to understand that there is a chance of a blood clot forming on the new valve or inside the heart chambers and that they will need to take long-term warfarin after the operation if the valve is metallic or for a few weeks if the valve is a tissue valve. Dose adjustment will involve regular blood tests, whether at the anticoagulant clinic of the local hospital or at the general practitioner's (GP's) surgery. It is also essential to ensure that the patient is aware they should not take any additional medications without either the doctor or the pharmacist being aware of this as the warfarin dose may require adjustment.

HEART TRANSPLANTATION

Heart transplantation may be an option for patients with end-stage severe heart failure, those whose heart failure is no longer effectively controlled by drug treatment and those whose heart is so severely damaged that they are at high risk of dying. With appropriate patient selection heart transplantation improves the chances of survival and may dramatically increase exercise capacity and quality of life.[5,6] Acute rejection is now less of a problem with modern immunosuppressive therapy, but the long-term outlook is more guarded because of transplant coronary artery disease and the longer term consequences of immunosuppression such as infection, hypertension, renal failure and malignancy.

However, only a limited number of transplants are done each year in this country, usually less than 300.

Not all patients are suitable for heart transplantation (see Table 5.1). Suitability will depend on:

1. the severity of the symptoms and estimated prognosis

2. co-morbidities including renal dysfunction

3. the patient's general health and psychological fitness.

Where a cardiological assessment identifies a patient suitable for a heart transplant, the patient will be referred to a transplant centre for a specialist assessment. Even then many patients do not require transplantation once their conventional medical therapy is optimized. Suitable candidates will be placed on a waiting list for a suitable heart: the number of transplants offered is severely limited by the availability of donor hearts.

The patient may be called at any time should a suitable heart become available. However, most people have to wait for approximately 6 months. Those with a serious condition may require hospitalization while waiting.

Following the operation, patients will generally remain in an intensive care unit for some time before being moved to a cardiac care unit. Immunosuppressant therapy will be given and will be continued in some form lifelong. Most patients are discharged 2–3 weeks after the operation, but will require several months convalescence before they get back to a normal way of life. Patients should be offered a place on a cardiac rehabilitation programme offering exercise and physiotherapy, as well as information about how to live with their new heart. They will also need to have specialist check-ups at regular intervals following discharge.

OTHER PROCEDURES

Some patients may require procedures for problems with their heart rhythm. These may include the use of an artificial pacemaker or an implantable cardiac defibrillator.

Table 5.1 Patients generally not considered suitable for heart transplantation

Patients who misuse alcohol or recreational drugs
Patients unable to cooperate
Patients with chronic, uncontrolled mental disease
Patients who have been treated for cancer within the previous 5 years
Patients with systemic disease with multi-organ involvement
Patients with uncontrolled infection
Patients with severe renal failure (creatinine clearance <50 ml/min) or serum creatinine >250 μmol/l
Patients who have recently had leg ulcers or deep vein thrombosis
Patients with an unhealed peptic ulcer
Patients with evidence of significant liver damage
Patients with other disease with a poor life expectancy

An artificial pacemaker may be fitted for patients with bradycardia due to, for example, sick sinus syndrome or heart block. Fitting a pacemaker will take approximately 1 h under a local anaesthetic, but it will usually require the patient to stay in hospital overnight and they will need regular pacemaker check-ups afterwards, usually every year. Generally, the pacemaker batteries last for 5–10 years before needing to be replaced.

Approximately one-third of patients with severe heart failure have conduction disturbances resulting in uncoordinated ventricular contraction. Multi-site pacing, whereby both ventricles are stimulated simultaneously and their contraction is programmed to occur at the optimal time after atrial contraction, has been shown to result in improved haemodynamics and an improvement in symptoms and exercise capacity. Whether this translates into long-term improvements in morbidity and mortality is currently the subject of several controlled studies, but preliminary evidence is encouraging.[7-10]

The use of an implantable cardiac defibrillator is likely to be appropriate in heart failure patients with recurrent ventricular tachycardia or fibrillation or 'failed' sudden death. The defibrillator monitors the heart rhythm and shocks the heart if it senses ventricular tachycardia or fibrillation, reverting the heart back to its normal rhythm. Fitting a defibrillator usually involves a stay in hospital of 2–3 days for the operation, which is usually carried out under a local anaesthetic. Implantable cardiac defibrillator therapy has been shown to improve survival in patients who have suffered a previous cardiac arrest or those with symptomatic ventricular arrhythmias and reduced systolic left ventricular function.[11-13] However, their role has not been studied in unselected populations of patients with heart failure and several morbidity and mortality studies are currently under way. An automatic implantable cardiac defibrillator can be combined with a dual chamber or multi-site pacemaker.

Mechanical support in the form of a left ventricular assist device may be required as a 'bridge' to transplantation for a severely sick heart failure patient. At present, such support usually relies on external blood pumps and is limited by infections or thromboembolic complications. Modern devices are implantable, although an external battery pack and subcutaneous induction coil are still required. Given the scarcity of donor hearts, some patients may require support for more than 1 year, suggesting a role for these devices as 'destination therapy', i.e. where transplantation is not going to take place. The Randomised Evaluation of Mechanical Assistance for Treatment of Chronic Heart Failure Study showed that implantation of a left ventricular assist device can improve survival in end-stage heart failure patients.[14] Further trials are currently under way.

Recently, transplantation of the first artificial heart was recorded in a patient with terminal heart failure. Further into the future, current research holds out the prospect of preventing and treating heart failure by means of cell and gene therapy, for instance by replacing diseased heart tissue with new myocytes. Such developments are still in their infancy. The use of genetically modified pig hearts as 'xenotransplants' remains several decades away, with public antipathy to research on genetically modified animals being a key factor in reducing the likelihood of this therapy being introduced.

Case Studies

A patient with angina

Sixty-eight-year-old Ronnie Holdsworth had a heart attack 8 years ago, which subsequently left him with mild angina. Four years ago he was diagnosed as having developed heart failure, which responded well to the introduction of diuretics, angiotensin-converting enzyme (ACE) inhibitors and beta blockade. Around a year ago he returned to his GP complaining of increasing angina, for which he was given a GTN spray. Recently, Ronnie noticed that he had been taking it much more frequently.

The GP checked his thyroid function tests and full blood count, both of which were normal. His electrocardiogram (ECG) showed that he had not developed atrial fibrillation. Although his heart failure syndrome was well controlled chest pain was the limiting factor. The GP added oral nitrates for a few weeks, which resulted in little improvement in his symptoms. He then prescribed amlodipine and reviewed the patient again. Ronnie was slightly better, but still found that he was unable to do his normal daily activities; occasionally he woke up at night with chest pain, which resolved with GTN spray.

The GP referred him to hospital where he was reviewed. It was clear that he had poor ventricular function, but the consultant said this did not preclude a bypass operation or angioplasty. Ronnie was scheduled for angiography with a view to intervention if the anatomy was appropriate.

Case Studies

A young patient with heart failure – transplantation

Following his flu-like illness last winter, 35-year-old Tony Groombridge was irritated by the fact that the cough never completely cleared up. Some weeks ago, finding himself increasingly breathless and with very swollen legs, he decided to consult his GP.

A series of investigations confirmed the GP's suspected diagnosis of heart failure: the ECG showed sinus rhythm and left bundle branch block and the chest X-ray showed a grossly enlarged heart with alveolar pulmonary oedema.

Tony was admitted to hospital immediately, where an echocardiogram showed a very dilated left ventricle with globally poor systolic function and moderate mitral regurgitation.

He was treated initially with diuretics and an ACE inhibitor, although this was not tolerated at high doses because of low blood pressure and deteriorating renal function. Tony's condition then deteriorated further until he required intravenous inotropic therapy. He also developed atrial fibrillation with further worsening of symptoms and was referred to the local heart transplantation centre, where he was assessed and placed on the list for the next available heart.

REFERENCES

1. Coronary Artery Surgery Study (CASS): a randomized trial of coronary artery bypass surgery. Quality of life in patients randomly assigned to treatment groups. *Circulation* 1983; **68**: 951–60.
2. Parisi AF, Folland ED, Hartigan P. A comparison of angioplasty with medical therapy in the treatment of single-vessel coronary artery disease. Veterans Affairs ACME Investigators. *N Engl J Med* 1992; **326**: 10–16.
3. Passamani E, Davis KB, Gillespie MJ, Killip T. A randomized trial of coronary artery bypass surgery: survival of patients with a low ejection fraction. *N Engl J Med* 1985; **312**: 1665–71.
4. Gibbons RJ, Chatterjee K, Daley J et al. ACC/AHA/ACP-ASIM guidelines for the management of patients with chronic stable angina: a report of the American College of Cardiology/American Heart Association Task Force on Practice Guidelines (Committee on Management of Patients With Chronic Stable Angina). *J Am Coll Cardiol* 1999; **33**: 2092–197.
5. Hosenpud JD, Bennett LE, Keck BM, Fiol B, Boucek MM, Novick RJ. The Registry of the International Society for Heart and Lung Transplantation: sixteenth official report – 1999. *J Heart Lung Transplant* 1999; **18**: 611–26.
6. Paris W, Woodbury A, Thompson S et al. Returning to work after heart transplantation. *J Heart Lung Transplant* 1993; **12**(Part 1): 46–53.
7. Cazeau S, Ritter P, Lazarus A et al. Multisite pacing for end-stage heart failure: early experience. *Pacing Clin Electrophysiol* 1996; **19**(Part2): 1748–57.
8. Auricchio A, Stellbrink C, Block M et al. Effect of pacing chamber and atrioventricular delay on acute systolic function of paced patients with congestive heart failure. The Pacing Therapies for Congestive Heart Failure Study Group. The Guidant Congestive Heart Failure Research Group. *Circulation* 1999; **99**: 2993–3001.
9. Cazeau S, Leclercq C, Lavergne T et al. Effects of multisite biventricular pacing in patients with heart failure and intraventricular

conduction delay. *N Engl J Med* 2001; **344**: 873–80.

10. Abraham WT. MIRACLE (Multisite In-synch Randomized Clinical Evaluation) Trial data. In *American College of Cardiology Meeting*, Orlando, FL, March 2001.

11. Moss AJ, Hall WJ, Cannom DS *et al.* Improved survival with an implanted defibrillator in patients with coronary disease at high risk for ventricular arrhythmia. Multicenter Automatic Defibrillator Implantation Trial Investigators. *N Engl J Med* 1996; **335**: 1933–40.

12. The antiarrhythmics versus implantable defibrillators. A comparison of antiarrhythmic-drug therapy with implantable defibrillators in patients resuscitated from near-fatal ventricular arrhythmias. *N Engl J Med* 1997; **337**: 1576–83.

13. Buxton AE, Lee KL, Fisher JD, Josephson ME, Prystowsky EN, Hafley G. A randomized study of the prevention of sudden death in patients with coronary artery disease. Multicenter Unsustained Tachycardia Trial Investigators. *N Engl J Med* 1999; **341**: 1882–90.

14. Rose EA, Gelijns AC, Moskowitz AJ *et al.* for the Randomized Evaluation of Mechanical Assistance for the Treatment of Congestive Heart Failure (REMATCH) Study Group. Long-term mechanical left ventricular assistance for end-stage heart failure. *N Engl J Med* 2001; **345**: 1435–43.

Chapter 6

Ongoing care of patients with heart failure

Patients with heart failure are often elderly and frail. Over time, most patients will experience increased symptoms. Therefore, once the diagnosis has been made and treatment instituted, a significant degree of ongoing monitoring by health care professionals is likely to be required.

In addition, heart failure is commonly associated with a reduced quality of life for the patient and often with increased levels of anxiety. Heart failure may have strongly negative connotations for patients, many of whom equate it with 'cardiac arrest'. Experience and feedback from patient and carer focus groups suggests that an early and frank discussion of the diagnosis and treatment options is greatly appreciated by patients.

Ideally, therefore, health care professionals should place great emphasis on the need for good communication with patients while remaining sensitive to the information needs of individual patients and tailoring the method and content of communications appropriately.

Where possible, discussions should seek to explain the nature of the disorder to the patient and, where appropriate, to explain basic cardiac physiology. This may help to reassure the patient and to empower them (and their carers) to take a more active role in their own management. Any anxieties the patient has should be explored. These may include issues relating to employment, driving and sexual function.

Essentially heart failure patients fall into two groups with regard to monitoring:

1. chronic, relatively stable heart failure

2. unstable, difficult to manage patients.

MONITORING PATIENTS WITH CHRONIC, RELATIVELY STABLE HEART FAILURE

Heart failure is a serious condition with an annual mortality rate of approximately 10% even in clinically stable patients. In general, a review should be conducted at least every 3–6 months in patients who are stable. Reviews may have to be much more frequent in other circumstances.

There should be an assessment of the patient's symptoms at each review looking for changes in their symptoms and severity (using, for example, the New York Heart Association (NYHA) classification). Discussion should probe the patient's ability to cope with their heart failure, their ability to get upstairs, do the shopping and housework and social factors. The physical examination should include blood pressure (taken with the patient lying down and then standing) and heart rate and rhythm, together with assessment of the patient's weight and any signs of fluid retention, which will require examining the jugular venous pressure, listening to the lungs and looking for dependent oedema such as ankle swelling. If there is any suspicion that their heart rhythm has changed or if there is any palpitation the patient should have a 12-lead electrocardiogram (ECG). Otherwise, assessment may be based on standard biochemical investigations such as urea and electrolytes and creatinine.

Derangements in biochemical parameters may be the result of the patient's drug therapy. Electrolyte disturbances are common in patients taking diuretics, but are rarely seen in patients with untreated heart failure, while concomitant administration of angiotensin-converting enzyme (ACE) inhibitors and potassium-sparing diuretics may lead to hyperkalaemia. Elevated serum creatinine may result from excessive treatment with diuretics and/or ACE inhibitors.

Further blood tests may also be required depending on the patient's other medications. For example, for those on amiodarone it is also important to check thyroid and liver function tests. It is important to remember that liver enzymes may be elevated by hepatic congestion. Consideration should be given to the patient's co-morbidities, the most usual being coronary artery disease, which will require a review of secondary prevention measures such as aspirin and statins, with measurement of serum cholesterol perhaps every 1–2 years. For those patients taking a statin, liver function tests should also be measured. Those taking warfarin, as many heart failure patients will be, should already be having regular blood tests to check for anticoagulation control. Change in medication, such as the addition of a short course of antibiotic for a chest infection, should trigger more frequent monitoring of anticoagulation control.

The review provides the opportunity for the doctor to reiterate previously given advice regarding lifestyle measures such as exercise, diet and advice on flu vaccination and travel, particularly in the summer period. In addition, the doctor should also review all medication with the patient in order to be satisfied with what the patient is taking and that the patient is complying with therapy and understands the need to do so. The general practitioner (GP) should always be on the look out for potential drug interactions, the most important being upset of warfarin by taking antibiotics or by medications purchased over the counter by the patient, such as non-steroidal anti-inflammatory drugs. These might impact on the patient's renal function and upset control of their heart failure syndrome.

The review can also allow clinicians to pick up a range of medical complications, including deep vein thrombosis as a result of immobility, gout due to diuretic therapy, and depression (which is common among heart failure patients and may be related to the impact of the symptoms on their daily activities of living). While depression should therefore improve with better symptom control, some patients will remain significantly clinically depressed and may require treatment. Antidepressant medication is generally avoided because of concerns regarding possible arrhythmias with tricyclic antidepressants and, where treatment is necessary, modern antidepressants such as the selective serotonin reuptake inhibitors are generally preferred. Other non-pharmacological approaches to depression, such as counselling, may prove useful.

Given sufficient and suitable education, some patients with chronic, relatively stable heart failure will be able to monitor their own heart failure, adjusting their diuretic dose in line with their weight and symptoms. However, this does not preclude the necessity for a regular medical review.

In an emergency...

All heart failure patients should know what to do in an emergency. They should be told that if they wake up at night extremely breathless they should call for an ambulance. However, even those with a stable illness may deteriorate and notice, for instance, an increase in weight or breathlessness for no apparent reason.

Therefore, all patients should have a contact point, whether it is the GP, a heart failure nurse specialist or a heart failure clinic, that they can contact in order to get their condition reviewed at the earliest possible opportunity. Without this, it is very likely that the patient will deteriorate quickly and require emergency admission to hospital.

Table 6.1   Checklist for monitoring patients with heart failure

Symptoms	Has the patient's NYHA class changed?
Signs	Have there been any changes in the patient's (1) blood pressure (lying down and standing), (2) heart rate and rhythm and (3) weight?
	Are there any signs of oedema?
Blood tests	Urea and electrolytes
	Creatinine
	Thyroid function tests if on amiodarone
	Liver function tests if on amiodarone
	Coagulation control for those on warfarin
Co-morbidities	Coronary artery disease
	Valvular disease
	Diabetes
Lifestyle management	Is the patient observing advice on (1) diet, (2) physical activity and (3) smoking?
Co-medications	Is the patient taking any other prescribed and/or proprietary medications?
Medical complications	Observe the patient for (1) angina or other symptoms of coronary artery disease, (2) deep vein thrombosis or (3) depression

MONITORING PATIENTS WITH UNSTABLE, DIFFICULT TO MANAGE HEART FAILURE

For unstable patients the key issue is when should they be referred to hospital. In general, this is necessary when a patient's heart failure fails to respond to medical therapy and is worsening or when therapy is changed. However, all of the following situations may trigger a referral.

• The patient is failing to gain control of fluid retention. Despite moderate doses of oral diuretics, the patient's weight is increasing and/or they are getting more breathless.

• The patient is waking up at night with marked breathlessness (paroxysmal nocturnal dyspnoea) despite oral diuretic therapy.

• The patient is hypotensive with symptoms (often more marked on change of posture) that do not settle down with adjustment of therapy by the GP.

• The patient is in pulmonary oedema (i.e. much more breathless than normal). This would indicate a need for an urgent referral.

• GP examination suggests significant new murmurs.

• GP investigation suggests a change in the patient's heart rhythm, for example a change from sinus rhythm to atrial fibrillation. It is always important to consider the patient's risk of thromboembolism and the need for anticoagulation.

• The patient is experiencing syncopal episodes. Syncope in a heart failure patient must be treated extremely seriously and discussed with the cardiologist as it may reflect life-threatening arrhythmia.

• When the patient has severe associated vascular disease. In particular, care is required before initiating ACE inhibitors in patients with co-existing renovascular disease.

• The patient and his or her carers have concerns about home management. Since many heart failure patients are elderly their cognitive function may not be as good as younger patients and the involvement of the principal carer or spouse is often vital.

In each of these situations there is a strong possibility that there will need to be a change in therapy or referral for other procedures or investigations and treatment.

For a patient in whom therapy is changed or a new therapy is initiated, the GP should arrange to see the patient more frequently. As in patients with stable heart failure, the important signs to be monitored are the control of symptoms, fluid retention, blood pressure and renal function. If the patient is taking warfarin then closer attention should be paid because of the possibility of the control of anticoagulation being upset by the new medication.

Practical considerations ...

The majority of patients who are on stable best therapy will remain stable and will require only routine review. This will require more time than the average primary care consultation if it is to be done properly: it is worth booking two slots instead of one for a review appointment. However, it is important that there is some mechanism by which changes in the patient's biochemistry are highlighted and acted upon. With drugs such as digoxin, which is still frequently used in clinical practice, it is important to look out for the symptoms and signs of digoxin toxicity such as nausea and vomiting and to allow time for measuring digoxin levels.

There are several models that may be appropriate for providing the ongoing care that heart failure patients need and specialized care provided within the context of a heart failure clinic is one model that has proven to be particularly useful.

SPECIALIZED CARE: THE HEART FAILURE CLINIC

Reducing morbidity and mortality from heart failure are important long-term goals, but improving the patient's quality of life is equally important.

Patients with heart failure are often frail and vulnerable. The condition can have devastating effects on patients' quality of life, particularly for a patient group that often has inadequate access to help and advice, which can reduce adherence with even the best management approaches.

Heart failure management can be complex, involving a multitude of health care professionals, including cardiologists, geriatricians, pharmacists and physiotherapists, psychologists, dietitians, social services, primary care physicians, district nurses and palliative care services.

In order to coordinate the complex care that patients may require, hospitals increasingly have a heart failure team in which the heart failure nurse specialist provides the pivotal link between the disparate members of this multidisciplinary group.

The heart failure nurse specialist can provide education to the patient and their carers about heart failure and its signs and symptoms. In addition, the nurse can discuss risk factors and lifestyle issues that may affect heart failure and how the illness may impact upon the patient's social activities or employment. The nurse can also provide information regarding the importance of influenza and pneumococcal vaccination.

Additional, specific roles of the specialist heart failure nurse may include the following.

- Undertaking physical examinations and ordering and interpreting blood tests and monitoring the patient's electrolyte balance and kidney function.

- Adjusting doses of specific drugs such as diuretics, ACE inhibitors and beta blockers within agreed management algorithms.

- Drawing up treatment and follow-up programmes tailored to the individual patient.

- Encouraging the patient to take an active role in managing their own disease, perhaps through the use of patient-held diaries for monitoring weight and symptoms such as dyspnoea, orthopnoea and nocturnal diuresis and for making appropriate adjustments in diuretic dosages.

- Early detection of deteriorating control of the patient's heart failure syndrome.

- Ensuring long-term adherence to treatment.

- Establishing a support network for each patient with
  other services as appropriate, such as physiotherapy,
  social services and palliative care services in more
  advanced cases.

The potential benefits are substantial, with reduced
hospital admission rates, improved quality of life and
lower costs. These benefits have now been demonstrated
in a considerable body of literature.

- Experienced heart failure physician and nurse teams
  have been shown to reduce hospitalization rates in
  patients with heart failure.[1]

- Nurse-led multidisciplinary intervention involving
  home visits has been shown to reduce hospital
  readmission rates, improve quality of life and reduce
  the costs of care.[2-4]

- Clinic-based follow-up of heart failure patients over
  12 months providing educational programmes that
  focus on treatment can lengthen the time to first
  readmission by one-third and also reduce the number
  of hospitalizations, length of hospitalization and
  costs of care.[5]

- Compared with usual care, home-based nurse
  intervention reduces the risk of death or hospitalization from heart failure by one-third.[6]

In primary care the provision of dedicated clinics has
improved the management of chronic conditions such as
asthma, diabetes and coronary heart disease. It is
reasonable to suppose that dedicated heart failure clinics,
whether hospital based or based within general practice,
run by a doctor or nurse with an interest and training in
heart failure have the potential to do the same for patients
with heart failure.

Such clinics offer the heart failure nurse the
opportunity of educating patients about their condition,
both through discussion and by the provision of written
materials particularly in relation to treatment and the role
that patients can play. Messages can be reinforced and

drug treatment simplified and rationalized where appropriate.

The close contact between the nurse and the patient and their carer(s) enables early identification of clinical deterioration and allows for prompt referral for specialist opinion.

END OF LIFE CARE

The aim of managing heart failure is to improve the quality of life for patients. For most patients, heart failure is still an incurable disease and for those patients approaching the end of life the principles of palliative care become important: that of improving the quality of dying for the patient and of its effects on the patient's family and carers.

There is not an extensive literature relating to palliative care in patients with heart failure. However, there has been a population-based retrospective survey of a random sample of people who died in 20 English health districts during 1990, which included 675 patients dying from heart disease.[7]

This Regional Study of Care for the Dying found that people dying from heart disease reported a wide range of distressing and prolonged symptoms, such as pain, dyspnoea, poor mood and anxiety. Many had symptoms equal in severity to those experienced by cancer patients, for whom it is accepted practice that they should be managed by specialist palliative care services. Yet few were able to obtain adequate information regarding their condition and its prognosis; too often doctors find it difficult to discuss death with their patients.[8]

Today it is increasingly accepted that patients with heart failure would benefit from input from specialist palliative care.

However, while the terminal phase of heart failure may be as bad as cancer both in terms of symptoms and distress, death in heart failure is often not signalled as clearly.[9]

Where decompensation results in hospital admission patients may recover to be discharged from hospital with improvement in their symptoms and functional class, while a relatively high proportion of all deaths in heart failure are sudden rather than involving a gradual deterioration in control.

In those patients in whom deterioration is gradual, a discussion about prognosis and the patient's and family's wishes is essential and should ideally be undertaken before the last days of life. There should be good communication between the GP and the family and also with secondary care. There is a good case for bringing in the palliative care team, or at least asking for advice.

A small retrospective study has suggested that specialist palliative care teams can apply generic palliative care skills to managing heart failure.[10] From the patient's viewpoint, it is essential to overcome communication difficulties and to provide psychological, spiritual and social support, symptom control, end of life care and subsequent bereavement support for carers.

Liaison with the palliative care team may be a particularly useful role for the specialist nurse.

Case Studies
How patients benefit from attending a heart failure clinic

Robert Bruce developed heart failure approximately 12 months ago and had diuretics and ACE inhibitors introduced by his GP before undergoing full assessment in the hospital heart failure clinic. At the clinic, the consultant examined him and decided he was a suitable candidate for beta blockade. Carvedilol was introduced by the nurse in the clinic and titrated upwards to 25 mg twice daily in fortnightly intervals.

Subsequently he attended the clinic for review every 3 months. At one recent appointment his weight had increased slightly, which was confirmed by the nurse on the scales. In conversation with Robert's wife the nurse scored the patient's symptoms using the NYHA scale and completed a quality of life questionnaire. She also took him for a 'walk test' in the hospital corridor. She found that Robert was becoming more breathless. His medication was reviewed and it was clear that there was good concordance with therapy, which his wife confirmed and that no new 'over-the-counter' drugs had been started.

The nurse followed a protocol for investigating patients like Robert. She checked his urea and electrolyte and creatinine levels, arranged thyroid function tests and performed an ECG. She also adjusted his dose of frusemide from 40 mg in the morning to 80 mg and arranged to review the patient 2 weeks later. Both Robert and his wife were given information on how he should monitor his weight and adjust his diuretic dose should there be any sign of decompensation.

Information was fed back by letter to the GP, who arranged alternate reviews with the heart failure clinic every 3 months. In the meantime, Robert was given a contact number to phone should he need urgent help.

Case Studies

How patients benefit from attending a heart failure clinic continued

Subsequently, Robert returned to the clinic with his weight back to normal and his breathlessness much improved. Although the patient and his wife had not previously discussed prognosis with the doctor, when they saw the nurse they were clearly concerned about whether he was likely to deteriorate again. She had a general discussion with them both about these issues and also informed both the GP and the cardiologist that it would be worthwhile raising these issues with Robert at his next appointment.

How end of life care can help patients and their carers

Ronald Stone was a 69-year-old man who had undergone a bypass operation 10 years earlier and had subsequent angina treated by angioplasty together with heart failure for the previous 4 years treated with a diuretic, ACE inhibitor and beta blockade. Over the previous 12 months he had required increasing doses of diuretics for controlling fluid retention. Some months ago he presented to his GP complaining of extreme lethargy and inability to undertake physical activity. The GP noticed he had a cachectic appearance and his history revealed that he had lost approximately 3.6 kg in the previous 3 months.

Examination showed that his full blood count was normal, while liver function tests revealed mildly reduced albumin and bilirubin. While heart failure may cause cachexia, other causes have first to be excluded. A range of other tests was also performed, including a chest X-ray, faecal occult blood tests and thyroid function tests. Since all of these tests were normal it was felt that cardiac failure was the cause of the patient's cachexia.

The GP consulted a cardiology specialist who told him that at present there were no proven therapies for cardiac cachexia, but that a number of experimental therapies had been investigated. After further discussion of the case, both doctors felt that it would be very important to communicate to the patient and his wife the cause of the weight loss, together with the fact that the heart failure was worsening and that there was a limit to what medical therapy could do for him.

Unsurprisingly the patient had many questions and asked bluntly whether he was dying. The doctors chose to be honest with him. They sought advice from a member of the local palliative care team, who arranged for the local hospice nurse to visit Ronald.

She was able to give him and his wife a great deal of helpful information and advice regarding nutritional supplements, gentle exercise and aids for the home, such as sheepskin rugs to guard against pressure sores. Through her discussions, she was able to help both Ronald and his wife prepare for his death.

The heart failure nurse specialist also continued to visit Ronald and his wife at home to help with his symptom control. Unfortunately, however, Ronald developed a chest infection and his condition rapidly deteriorated. He was admitted to the hospice over a weekend, rapidly losing consciousness. He died within 24 h. Although she was understandably upset, Ronald's wife later said that she was better able to cope with his death by having been prepared for it in his last few months by the various health care professionals who visited him.

REFERENCES

1. McAlister FA, Lawson FME, Teo KK, Armstrong PW. A systematic review of randomized trials of disease management programs in heart failure. *Am J Med* 2001; **110**: 378–84.
2. Rich MW, Beckham V, Wittenberg C *et al.* A multidisciplinary intervention to prevent the readmission of elderly patients with congestive heart failure. *N Engl J Med* 1995; **333**: 1190–5.
3. Stewart S, Vandenbroek AJ, Pearson S, Horowitz JD. Prolonged beneficial effects of a home-based intervention on unplanned readmissions and mortality among patients with congestive heart failure. *Arch Intern Med* 1999; **159**: 257–61.
4. Stewart S, Marley JE, Horowitz JD. Effects of a multidisciplinary, home-based intervention on unplanned readmissions and survival among patients with chronic congestive heart failure: a randomised controlled study. *Lancet* 1999; **354**: 1077–83.
5. Cline CMJ, Israelsson BYA, Willenheimer RB *et al.* A cost effective management programme for heart failure reduces hospitalisation. *Heart* 1998; **80**: 442–6.
6. Blue L, Lang E, McMurray JJV *et al.* Randomised controlled trial of specialist nurse intervention in heart failure. *BMJ* 2001; **323**: 715–18.
7. McCarthy M, Lay M, Addington HJ. Dying from heart disease. *J R Coll Phys Lond* 1996; **30**: 325–8.
8. McCarthy M, Addington-Hall JM, Ley M. Communication and choice in dying from heart disease. *J R Soc Med* 1997; **90**: 128–31.
9. Hockley JM, Dunlop R, Davies RJ. Survey of distressing symptoms in dying patients and their families in hospital and the response to a symptom control team. *BMJ* 1988; **296**: 1715–17.
10. Thorns AR, Gibbs LM, Gibbs JS. Management of severe heart failure by specialist palliative care. *Heart* 2001; **85**: 93.

Chapter 7

Audits and standards in heart failure

As the previous chapters have demonstrated, growing understanding of the pathophysiology of heart failure has led to considerable improvements in treatment based on therapies for improving survival and hospitalization rates that have been proven in clinical trials. In addition, the greater focus on the multidisciplinary approach to follow-up has been shown to reduce hospital readmission.

However, there is little evidence that recent years have seen the significant improvement in the prognosis of patients with heart failure that might have been expected. Readmission rates for heart failure also remain depressingly high.

There are many factors that may contribute to the poor outcomes among patients with heart failure. These include

- poor compliance with treatment

- adverse effects from treatment

- inadequate education of patients regarding management of their disease

- inadequate contact with appropriately trained health care professionals.

One further factor likely to have contributed to this situation is poor implementation of the available evidence base by health care professionals.

Despite the availability of many guidelines for the diagnosis and management of heart failure, many patients continue to receive suboptimal treatment. In particular, angiotensin-converting enzyme (ACE) inhibitors are often not prescribed to patients or are prescribed in doses lower than those shown to be beneficial in large-scale clinical trials.[1-4] This situation is even worse with respect to the use of beta blockers.

Most health care professionals are keen to ensure that the care they provide to their patients is evidence based. In addition, many health care professionals are keen to know how their performance compares with that of colleagues elsewhere. Clinical audit, that is the systematic assessment of the quality of care against recognized professional standards, provides a means by which this aim can be achieved within general practice. In order to complete the audit cycle any discrepancy should be examined and measures taken to rectify shortcomings, with the situation reviewed again subsequently.

HOW TO CONDUCT A HEART FAILURE AUDIT IN GENERAL PRACTICE

Discuss the audit among members of the primary health care team and nominate a coordinator for the project. The team members should also agree on the aims of the audit and the process by which data will be collected and analysed.

Areas relating to the care of heart failure patients that are suitable for audit in primary care include the following.

Diagnosis.

- How many patients in the practice have a diagnosis of heart failure?
- Have all patients with heart failure had an echocardiogram to assess left ventricular function?

Treatment.

- Are all patients with confirmed heart failure taking an ACE inhibitor (unless there is a documented contraindication)?
- Have ACE inhibitor doses been increased where possible to those used in the large clinical trials?

Monitoring treatment and ongoing care.

- Were blood pressure and renal function recorded before and after the start of ACE inhibitors?
- How many patients on ACE inhibitors have had their urea and electrolyte levels measured in the past year?
- Have all patients with heart failure had an influenza and/or one-off pneumococcal vaccination?

The first step is to identify the practice notes of all heart failure patients in the target group. This may be achieved by means of a disease register, computer records (identifying patients using National Health Service (NHS) Read codes) (see Table 7.1) or even the repeat prescribing list (in order to identify those patients taking drugs such as diuretics and ACE inhibitors) (see Table 7.2).

A suitable sample size and sampling technique should be selected and a reasonable time-scale agreed for completion of the data collection and analysis.

Each set of notes should be studied or a computer search performed in order to determine the presence or absence of the required data, which should then be transferred onto a spreadsheet.

Table 7.1   Disease categories that may be associated with heart failure including standard NHS Read codes

Category	NHS Read code
Elderly >75 years old	R200
Confirmed congestive heart failure	G580
Symptomatic congestive heart failure	G580
Left ventricular dysfunction	G581-3/33BA
Recent myocardial infarction	323
Hypertension (essential)	G20
Ischaemic heart disease	G3
Atrial fibrillation	G5730
Heart valve disease	G54Z5
High cholesterol	44P3/44P4
Asthma/Coronary artery disease	H33/H32
Diabetes	C10
Chronic alcoholism	E231

Actual performance should then be compared with the accepted standards. Review of the information should then allow the team to determine whether the standards have been met.

A subsequent meeting of the primary health care team should discuss the results and decide what changes are

Table 7.2   Medicines that heart failure patients may be taking for heart failure, hypertension, coronary heart disease, post-myocardial infarction and arrhythmia

ACE inhibitors	captopril, cilazapril, enalapril, fosinopril, imidapril, lisinopril, perindopril, quinapril, ramipril and trandolapril
Beta blockers	acebutolol, atenolol, betaxolol, bisoprolol, carvedilol, celiprolol, esmolol, labetolol, metoprolol, nadolol, nebivolol, oxprenalol, pindolol, propranolol, sotalol and timolol
Calcium channel blockers	amlodipine, diltiazem, felodipine, isradipine, lacidipine, lercanidipine, nicardipine, nifedipine, nisoldipine and verapamil
Angiotension II receptor blockers	candesartan, eprosartan, irbesartan, losartan, telmisartan and valsartan
α_1-Antagonists	doxazosin, indoramin, phentolamine, prazosin and terazosin
Class I anti-arrhythmics	disopyramide, flecainide, mexiletine, propafenone, phenytoin, procainamide and quinidine
Central acting α-agonists	clonidine, methyldopa and moxonidine
Diuretics	amiloride, bendrofluazide, bumetanide, chlorthalidone, cyclopenthiazide, frusemide, hydrochlorothiazide, indapamide, metolazone, polythiazide, spironolactone, torasemide, triamterene and xipamide
Fibrates	bezafibrate, ciprofibrate, fenofibrate and gemfibrozil
Statins	atorvastatin, fluvastatin, pravastatin and simvastatin
Other drugs	adenosine, alprostadil, amiodarone, aminophylline, aspirin, cholestyramine, colestipol, diazoxide, digoxin, dobutamine, dopexamine, enoximone, glyceryl trinitrate, guanethidine, hydralazine, indomethacin, isoprenaline, isosorbide dinitrate, isosorbide mononitrate, metaraminol, minoxidil, nicorandil and theophylline

necessary for enabling the team to comply with the selected guidelines. The agreed changes should then be monitored and the audit cycle completed after a suitable time lapse.

PROFESSIONAL GUIDANCE

A number of professional bodies provide guidance on audits of the care of patients with heart failure. As yet in England and Wales there is no form of national audit for heart failure. However, the *National Service Framework for Coronary Heart Disease* urges primary care professionals to undertake an annual audit of the care they provide for people with heart failure (see Table 7.3).[5] This is likely to be updated by the National Institute for Clinical Excellence when it publishes its guidelines for the management of chronic heart failure in 2003.

In Scotland the Scottish Programme for Improving Clinical Effectiveness in Primary Care (SPICE-PC) has produced a 13-point audit package for the diagnosis and management of heart failure due to left ventricular dysfunction in patients with ischaemic heart disease, which is the most common cause of heart failure (see

Table 7.3   National Service Framework for Coronary Heart Disease: suggested audit topics

1.	The number and percentage of the registered population with a diagnosis of heart failure
2.	The number and percentage of people with confirmed heart failure or left ventricular dysfunction currently prescribed an ACE inhibitor
3.	The number and percentage of patients with a diagnosis of heart failure who have ever undergone echocardiography by practice and PCG/PCT
4.	Age–Sex standardized admission rates for heart failure by PCG/PCT and Health Authority
5.	Age–Sex standardized mortality rates for people with heart failure/left ventricular dysfunction
6.	The number and percentage of people with heart failure for whom specialist palliative care advice has been sought by practice and PCG/PCT

Table 7.4) (http://www.ceppc.org/spice/pdf/lvd.PDF).[6] It
has been distributed to every practice, primary care trust
and local health care council in Scotland.

Table 7.4 SPICE-PC criteria

1.	Practices will have a database that records cardiac failure: there will be a system in place for adding new patients to the database and the detection of defaulters from follow-up
2.	Patients with newly suspected heart failure will have a 12-lead electrocardiogram (ECG)
3.	Patients with newly suspected heart failure will have an echocardiogram if the ECG is abnormal and patients with existing clinically diagnosed heart failure will have had an echocardiogram at some time in the past if possible
4.	Patients with suspected heart failure will have a full blood count, biochemical profile (urea and electrolytes and liver function tests), blood glucose and thyroid function test and cholesterol evaluation
5.	Patients with suspected heart failure will have a medication review at diagnosis (including drugs known to worsen heart failure)
6.	Patients with heart failure will be treated with an ACE inhibitor unless contraindicated or unless there are significant side-effects
7.	Patients on ACE inhibitors for heart failure will be stabilized on recommended therapeutic doses
8.	Patients with heart failure will be prescribed a diuretic if there are symptoms or signs of fluid retention
9.	Patients with heart failure will be reviewed yearly at a minimum by an appropriately trained member of the primary care team: areas to be covered include clinical status and medication review
10.	Patients with heart failure will have their biochemistry checked at a minimum every year
11.	Patients with heart failure will receive an annual influenza vaccine unless there is specific contraindication
12.	Patients with heart failure will receive a one-off pneumococcal vaccine unless there is specific contraindication
13.	Patients who smoke tobacco should be advised and offered support to stop

Case Studies

How patients benefit when general practitioners audit their heart failure practice

At a practice meeting of the health centre it was decided that, in the current climate of clinical governance, it should undertake a prospective audit of its patients with confirmed or suspected heart failure.

A meeting of the practice team was convened and a project leader nominated to lead discussion of the audit process and its objectives. The roles of the team members were identified as follows.

- General practitioners: overseeing the audit standards, reviewing treatments and confirming management decisions.
- Practice manager: coordinating the audit with the project leader, planning the programme, identifying suitable patients using patients' records and analysing the data.
- Practice nurse: identifying patients from new patient screenings and from those attending other practice clinics and arranging for home-bound patients (including those in residential and nursing homes) to join the programme even though they may be unable to attend the surgery.
- Receptionist: identifying suitable patients when they make appointments or collect repeat prescriptions and flagging patients' notes and repeat prescriptions.

The team decided that it would adopt the European Society of Cardiology guidelines as its 'gold standard'. Initially, it set three audit standards.

1. That 80% of heart failure patients would be receiving an ACE inhibitor.
2. That 80% of all eligible heart failure patients would be offered treatment with a beta blocker.
3. To reduce the number of deaths from heart failure to no more than 5% at 12 months.

It was agreed that, at each patient visit, those with confirmed or suspected heart failure would be asked about symptoms such as dyspnoea, orthopnoea, oedema and paroxysmal nocturnal dyspnoea. These would be assessed and graded according to severity. The patient would also be asked about cardiac symptoms such as angina and about aspects of their diet, alcohol consumption, smoking habits and so on. Risk factor advice should be given as necessary.

The clinical examination would focus on the patient's weight and cardiovascular system, such as blood pressure, cholesterol level and blood glucose control. Importantly, the patient's medication would be reviewed, using questions probing whether they were taking their tablets regularly and whether they had experienced any side-effects. Doses might be adjusted in order to control blood pressure and minimize the signs and symptoms of heart failure and to maximize compliance.

All of these data, together with data on hospitalizations, referrals and deaths, were to be recorded in a patient record sheet such that at regular intervals the audit coordinator would be able to capture all of the data to present an overall picture of heart failure care within the practice and to compare the aggregated totals with the standards set for the practice at the outset.

Over the first year of the audit, the practice found that simply recording and feeding back information on how it managed its patients enabled it to meet the target for ACE inhibitor usage and to increase the number of patients given a trial of beta blockade even though it was unable to meet this target. In part this was due to a lack of sufficiently trained staff for administering beta blockers and titrating patients' dosages. At the team meeting called to discuss the audit results, it was decided that an approach should be made to the local hospital with a view to developing a shared care protocol for the management and treatment of patients with heart failure. It was felt that patients would benefit hugely from the expertise of the hospital's nurse-led heart failure clinic, which would also be able to train the practice staff in the use of these drugs.

Figure 7.1   Summary of the audit process

Arrange team quarterly team meetings to discuss heart failure, plan a clinical audit and and discuss the results

---

▼

Agree team members' roles and responsibilities, and agree a starting date for the audit as well as the audit period

---

▼

Set the targets for the heart failure outcomes to be monitored

---

▼

Identify all patients with and those at high risk of heart failure

---

▼

Classify patients into:
a) confirmed heart failure
b) suspected (but not confirmed) heart failure
c) high risk of future heart failure

▼

Prepare a patent register for each group

▼

Select a group to audit and enrol patients in the audit, following any local protocols regarding patent consent. Flag the patient's notes or computer record

---

▼

At the baseline and all subsequent visits:
a) record all the relevant data in the patient record sheet (which should be kept with the notes)
b) Follow the practice heart failure management and treatment guidelines

---

▼

At the end of each audit period, transfer all data from the patient record sheets and the registers into the chosen data capture format

---

▼

Analyse the data, comparing it with the targets set and plan improvements resetting the targets as necessary.

Continue to audit these patients, adding in other groups of heart failure patients as appropriate

REFERENCES

1. Bungard TJ, McAlister FA, Johnson JA, Tsuyuki RT. Underutilisation of ACE inhibitors in patients with congestive heart failure. *Drugs* 2001; **61**: 2021–33.

2. Stafford RS, Saglam D, Blumenthal D. National patterns of angiotensin-converting enzyme inhibitor use in congestive heart failure. *Arch Intern Med* 1997; **157**: 2460–4.

3. Clarke KW, Gray D, Hampton JR. Evidence of inadequate investigation and treatment of patients with heart failure. *Br Heart J* 1994; **71**: 584–7.

4. Mair FS, Crowley TS, Bundred PE. Prevalence, aetiology and management of heart failure in general practice. *Br J Gen Pract* 1996; **46**: 77–9.

5. Department of Health. *National Service Framework for Coronary Heart Disease: Modern Standards and Service Models.* London: Department of Health; 2000.

6. *Scottish Programme for Improving Clinical Effectiveness in Primary Care (SPICE-PC). Diagnosis and Management of Heart Failure Due to Left Ventricular Dysfunction in Patients with Ischaemic Heart Disease.* Available at www.ceppc.org.

Alphabetical index

Indexer: Dr Laurence Errington

Abreviations: CHD, coronary heart disease; HF, heart failure; LV, left ventricle; LVD, left ventricular dysfunction; MI, myocardial infarction.

signs of HF, 1, 18-19
in history-taking, 21
in monitoring checklist, 81
skeletal muscle abnormalities in chronic
HF, 10
smoking, 36
sodium retention
lifestyle ameliorating, 34-5
treatment, 44
South East Asians, aetiology of HF, 7
specialist opinion, referral, see referral
specialized care, 83-6
see also clinic
SPICE-PC, 94-5
spironolactone, 46, 54-5, 93
side-effects, 55
in treatment algorithm for LVD, 44
standards, 90-8
statins, 93
steroids, parenteral, 65
surgery (and invasive procedures), 30,
70-7
valvular disease, 18, 70, 71-2
survival
in HF, 11-13
in MI, improved, 4
Survival Trial of Antiarrhythmic Therapy
in Congestive HF, 57
sympathetic nervous system, 10
symptoms of HF, 1, 18-19
quality of life impact of, 5, 84
syncopal episodes, 82
systolic LV dysfunction, 1
treatment
algorithms, 44, 50
digoxin use, 56
diuretic use, cautions, 45
systolic LV function, measurement in
echocardiography, 24-5

tachycardia in history-taking, 21
telmisartan, 51, 93

terminal care, see end of life care
thiazide diuretics, 45
thromboembolism, previous, patients with,
59-60
thrombus, intracardiac, anti-thrombotic or
antiplatelet agents, 60
thyrotoxicosis, HF with atrial fibrillation
in, 27
TNF-α, see tumour necrosis factor-α
torasemide, 45, 93
transplantation
artificial heart, 75
heart, 70, 72-3
case study, 76
criteria for suitability/unsuitability,
72, 73
travelling abroad, 38-9
treatment, see management
triamterene, 46
tricyclic antidepressants, care
with/avoidance of, 65, 80
tumour necrosis factor-α, 11, 62-3
suppression (incl. receptor blockers),
62-3
12-lead ECG, 22-3

ultrasound, cardiac, see
echocardiography
urinalysis, 27

vaccination, 39
ValHeFT trial, 52
valsartan, 51, 52, 93
valvular disease, 8
treatment, 18, 63-4, 70, 71-2
vascular disease, severe associated, 82
vasoactive peptides, 10
vasodilator agents, 46-9, 58-9
vasopeptidase inhibitors, 62
venous pressure, jugular, 21
ventricular arrhythmias, 8
ventricular assist device, left, 74-5